YOUR FUTURE AS A CHIROPRACTOR

YOUR FUTURE AS A CHIROPRACTOR

By
G. HOWARD POTEET
and
MICHAEL A. PETTI

THE ROSEN PUBLISHING GROUP
New York

Published in 1977, 1984 by the Rosen Publishing Group
29 East 21st Street, New York, N.Y. 10010

Revised Edition 1984

Library of Congress Cataloging in Publication Data
Poteet, G   Howard.
    Your future as a chiropractor.

    Bibliography: p.
    1. Chiropractic—Vocational guidance.   I. Petti,
Michael A., joint author.   II. Title.
RZ236.P67   615'.534'023   77–8150
ISBN 0–8239–0383–4
Manufactured in the United States of America

Photograph: Courtesy of Palmer College of Chiropractic

About the Authors

DR. G. HOWARD POTEET has had a lifelong interest in the health care professions and in researching opportunities for young people to increase personal income.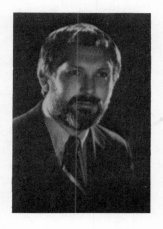
He received his doctorate from Teachers College, Columbia University, and he is Professor of English at Essex County College in Newark, New Jersey. In addition, he is Adjunct Professor at The University of Sarasota in Sarasota, Florida, where he serves as adviser to doctoral candidates.
Dr. Poteet is the author of twenty-four books, numerous articles, poems, and short stories. Some of his works have dealt with the sociology and psychology of subjects of interest to health care professionals.

Other works have concerned a wide range of job opportunities and careers. He is the editor and publisher of the newsletter "How to Make Extra Money." Dr. Poteet also has written an internationally syndicated series on ways to increase one's income.

A member of numerous professional organizations, Professor Poteet is listed in such directories as *Current American Authors, Who's Who in Computers and Automation, International Dictionary of Biography, Men of Achievement, International Dictionary of Authors and Writers,* and *Who's Who in the East.*

He and his wife, Frances, a children's librarian in Newark, New Jersey, have a daughter, Jennifer.

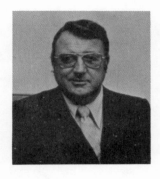 DR. MICHAEL A. PETTI is Associate Dean of Health Professions at Essex County Hospital, New Jersey, and holds the rank of Assoicate Professor of Neurology at Columbia Institute of Chiropractic, educational posts which he reached through an unusual route. Born in Newark, he attended high school there and was then signed by the Brooklyn Dodgers professional baseball team, with which he played for three years. After serving in the United States Air Force, he attended Seton Hall University, from which he received a B.S. degree in Business Administration and another certification in the field of teaching. He then entered Rutgers University and New York University, taking courses in real estate appraising. Thereafter, Dr. Petti abruptly changed course and took a doctorate degree in the field of Chiropractic at Columbia Institute of Chiropractic, where he was subsequently named Chairman of the Anatomy Department and was the recipient of the Distinguished Neurology Award. Currently, he has completed course work for the degree of Doctor of Education in Intercultural Education at Rutgers University and is preparing to write his dissertation.

Dr. Petti is extremely active in civic affairs. He has served three consecutive terms as Vice-President of the Newark Board of Education and is currently a member of the Newark Board of School Estimate. He serves on the Newark Advisory Council and the Health Manpower Committee of the Hospital and Health Planning Council of New Jersey, and collaborates with the Allied Health Program Development and Administration of the College of Medicine and Dentistry of New Jersey.

Contents

Preface

Do you enjoy helping others? Does lessening human suffering and making another's life easier appeal to you? If you answer "Yes" to those questions, you should consider Chiropractic as a career choice. Chiropractic is a service-oriented profession dedicated to improving the quality of life. The rewards for providing such a service go well beyond what can be measured in a bank account. Personal fulfillment, satisfaction, recognition, and the grateful smiles of thanks from your patients and their families will come your way as well. Such a calling is not for everyone and is indeed for only a select few. But certainly, trying to assist in the evolution of a better world through healthier individuals is a goal of the highest order. A chiropractor strives to achieve this every time he or she places a hand upon a patient's body.

The hallmark of chiropractic is the use of the hands to adjust, or change, another person. Chiropractors contend that aberrant function is the result of abnormal structure and that changing the abnormal structure causes an alteration in function. Chiropractic utilizes this concept of structure determining function to improve health. The wondrous harmony of body parts can easily be disrupted by one poorly functioning organ. Particularly with today's problems of pollution, radiation, and our own shortsightedness, chiropractic is a welcome addition to the health-care field. Often before symptoms are apparent, a chiropractic examination can reveal a structural disturbance, and appropriate adjustment of the spinal column can be begun. With proper training, virtually everyone can master chiropractic techniques that will enable them to contribute to easing life's stresses and strains for their patients.

A visit to a chiropractor's office or a school of chiropractic would be advised after you have read this book. Such a contact can provide a more personal and practical association with the profession. And since chiropractors are in the business of helping, you're sure to be welcomed.

Chiropractic today is in the mainstream of a revolution in health care. Olympic teams are actively using our services in an attempt to limit injuries and improve performance. The scope of practice is ever widening and ranges from the traditional spinal manipulation to acupuncture. Nutritional and dietary advice is becoming ever more popular as advances are made in research of various health-related problems. Cooperation between chiropractic and the other health-related professions is on the increase, and with research and development a priority in the profession, this trend is certain to continue. A holistic approach to health care is the wave of the future, and chiropractic is cresting with the wave.

There is no doubt of the necessity for well-trained medical personnel in the future of health-care services. Their contributions have been enormous and unquestionably will continue to be. However, much of the emphasis has been on intervening in crises. The question of why we get sick, not how or how to reverse the process, is at the root of today's health movement. It seems that everyone is involved in one form of exercise or another. Health clubs and spas are opening up everywhere. Bookstores, supermarkets, and television are flooded with the latest diet and exercise materials. All to what end? To keep our most valuable possession, our health. Chiropractic's unique and beautifully simple approach places it squarely in line with this goal.

The secrets of the human body are gradually unfolding through the efforts of chiropractic research. The complex interrelationships of the body systems are being unraveled and noninvasive "hands on" procedures developed. Society will no longer tolerate the proliferation of unnecessary surgery and high-risk experiments with human guinea pigs. Acupuncture and meridian therapy are today being taught side by side with the more traditional techniques involving moving vertebrae. New diagnostic methods are emerging as a means of guiding skilled hands to the proper location. Treatment of various ailments may require the use of adjunctive modalities such as ultrasound, electrical muscle stimulation, diathermy, and others.

Formerly, chiropractors shunned all forms of medication. Many considered chiropractic a "drugless" profession. Now, with the increased use of dietary guidance and glandular supplements, that term has been dropped. If you are interested in nutrition, chiropractic provides a fine avenue for its application. Today's high potencies and vast numbers of combination vitamin and mineral preparations require that we treat them as drugs. Chiropractic is not a panacea for all of our ills, in spite of new developments and broadening of the scope of practice. No chiropractor performs flawlessly; we are only human too. But we are trying, and new understanding of disease processes and nutritional deficiencies are being discovered daily and incorporated into our body of knowledge. Sophisticated kinesiological analyses and muscle testing are being done. Every available means possible for one human to assist another is under investigation. From the hair of our heads to the soles of our feet, researchers are exploring for better ways to alleviate suffering and misery. There is still plenty of room for pioneers in the chiropractic profession, and always will be!

Probably one of the most exciting new applications for chiropractic is the field of sports medicine. Professional teams, ballet companies, and the like are discovering the benefits of chiropractic. A thorough understanding of the body's biomechanics and the workings of joints, ligaments, and muscles makes chiropractic a natural for this burgeoning field. Truly, the future looks bright for this young profession. Even the inclusion of hospital privileges appears on the not too distant horizon.

Paul Ravener, D.C.

The Chiropractic Oath

I do hereby affirm before God and these assembled witnesses that I will keep this oath and stipulation.

To hold in esteem and respect those who taught me the chiropractic healing art; to follow the methods of treatment which according to my ability and judgment I consider for the benefit of my patients; to abstain from whatever is deleterious and mischievous; to stand ready at all times to serve my fellowman without distinction of race, creed, or color.

With purity I will pass my life and practice my art; I will at all times consider the patients under my care as of supreme importance; I will not spare myself in rendering them help which I have been taught to give by my alma mater; I will keep inviolate all things revealed to me as a physician.

While I continue to keep this oath unviolated, may it be granted to me to enjoy life and the practice of the chiropractic healing art, respected by all men at all times.

Adopted by the Council of Chiropractic Education
January 1972

CHAPTER I

What Is Chiropractic?

There are three major schools in the healing-arts profession: chiropractic, medicine, and osteopathy. Of the three, the youngest and fastest growing is chiropractic. It is also often the most misunderstood.

Chiropractic practitioners diagnose and treat human ailments without using drugs or surgery. Instead, chiropractic physicians use manipulation of the spine, clinical nutrition, and instruction in hygiene in providing health care to their patients.

Chiropractic is the largest drugless healing profession in the world. Its practitioners believe that man was created to be healthy and that his innate intelligence attempts to coordinate and control his bodily functions to maintain that balanced state of health. Chiropractic teaches that man is a part of nature and should therefore try to harmonize his life with nature.

Doctors of Chiropractic believe that illness results from the spinal vertebrae becoming misaligned, thus pinching a nerve and interfering with the natural state of health. If these vertebrae are adjusted back to their original position, the body will repair or adapt itself and health will be restored.

Chiropractors attempt to relieve pain and suffering by correcting the subluxation (the displaced spinal bone) through the use of skills and techniques learned in chiropractic college.

3

Make no mistake about it, the practice of chiropractic, like all professions, is often complex and difficult. But as its practitioners will tell you, it is highly rewarding and fulfilling.

The chiropractor works on a one-to-one basis with his patients, carefully and patiently explaining the reasons for the patient's illness, and sets up a program for his recovery.

The chiropractor makes few house calls; he treats almost all of his patients in his office. The equipment used in his profession is not portable, and thus the patient must come to him.

Generally the chiropractor practices alone in his own office. Currently, chiropractic is not utilized in the armed services nor in general hospitals; however, a chiropractor may treat patients in a private or industrial clinic or in a chiropractic hospital.

The Spears Free Clinic and Hospital for Poor Children, in Denver, Colorado, is the first and largest chiropractic hospital in the world. According to the hospital staff, Spears receives cases that are too advanced or too complicated for office treatment, cases requiring twenty-four-hour observation, cases needing more variety and frequency of treatment than is obtainable in office visits, and cases in which chiropractic and supplementary methods are available only at the hospital.

Chiropractic has been a center of controversy, and you should understand some points about those criticisms. For example, critics have often tried to disprove the value of chiropractic care by using reports of erroneous diagnosis or treatment for the wrong illness by chiropractors. To the fair-minded observer, this criticism is unjust. None of the healing arts is an exact science. There have been mistakes, unfortunately, in medical and osteopathic treatment as well as in chiropractic. For example, there was the tragedy in the 1960's caused by the distribution of thalidomide—a drug that produced deformities in newborn infants. Medical doctors have made faulty diagnoses, sewn up instruments inside patients after surgery, or made other serious errors in judgment. This is not to justify these errors, but to point out that they do occur.

Like medical and osteopathic practitioners, chiropractors have not always been successful in treating illnesses, and sad to say, poorly trained practitioners—as in all the health-care services— have made mistakes. Patients have come to realize that there are no guarantees, but most health-care professionals would rather be judged on their successes than on their failures. In modern times failures are the exception, so much so that they often make the headlines.

The volume of evidence showing the success of chiropractic care is increasing. Until recently practically no funds were available for chiropractic research, but this is gradually changing. A recent study reported in the respected medical magazine *Lancet* compared the effectiveness of medical and chiropractic care of 232 patients with back trouble. Dr. Robert L. Kane and his associates at the University of Utah College of Medicine found that patients were slightly more pleased by their improvement and with the care given them by chiropractors. Even though the chiropractors did only slightly better than medical doctors in this study, the research seems to indicate that chiropractic care is effective. There is no question that millions of people have found relief from pain and discomfort through the health care given by chiropractors. Future research may prove this success to the skeptical by the use of similar scientific statistical methods.

The training given to chiropractors has sometimes been the subject of criticism. Chiropractors agree that, because chiropractic is a recent science, in some instances training has left much to be desired. But this is true of the history of medical training as well. At the turn of the century dentists often taught themselves or apprenticed themselves to a practicing dentist. Medical colleges were not carefully regulated until the 1930's.

The profession of chiropractic and in particular the national associations such as the American Chiropractic Association (ACA) and the International Chiropractic Association (ICA) have shown intense interest in improving the quality of education of chiropractic physicians.

In 1974 the U.S. Office of Education set up an accrediting agency to evaluate the quality of colleges of chiropractic. Those colleges that are certified by the Council on Chiropractic Education offer a fully accredited doctoral degree. Graduates of such schools who pass the licensing examination are legally qualified to practice chiropractic.

Much of the criticism of chiropractic has come from the American Medical Association (AMA). This is because of a basic disagreement among health-care professionals on certain fundamental issues. Animosities have lessened over the years, however, as chiropractic colleges have tightened training requirements and evidence of chiropractic effectiveness is being gathered through carefully controlled research studies.

You will have to examine the evidence and decide for yourself whether chiropractic is what its advocates say.

The Beginning of the Art, Science, and
Philosophy of Chiropractic

In 1895, the same year that Wilhelm Roentgen discovered X-rays, Daniel David Palmer of Davenport, Iowa, restored the hearing of Harvey Lilliard, a janitor, by pressing a large bump above the fourth cervical vertebra. Lilliard said that seventeen years earlier he had bent over while working, heard something pop, and lost his hearing. Following Palmer's adjustment of the man's back, he was able to hear noises from the street instantly and his hearing gradually returned to normal.

"D. D.," as Dr. Palmer was called, began experimenting with the technique that he had discovered and met with success in treating his patients. He named the new method "chiropractic" from the Greek words meaning "done by hand."

B. J. Palmer, his son, developed the original concepts and ideas that his father had discovered and began teaching them in chiropractic schools, beginning around 1905. Like his father, (he advocated the adjustment of vertebrae to cure illness. His followers, however, sometimes used techniques borrowed from the other healing arts in their work.

To understand the development of chiropractic, you need to know a little about the history of health care. In the late 1890's health care was provided by a variety of practitioners—many of whom were outright quacks—with wide and diverse opinions on what caused illnesses. There were water cures, electric cures, and other techniques of dubious value. Patent medicines that promised to cure almost any kind of illness were advertised and sold. Hospitals were places where incurable patients went to die.

It is difficult for us today to realize how common epidemics were, how high the infant mortality was, and how little chance people had of achieving good health because of poor nutrition and inadequate sanitation.

It was in this milieu that the three basic health-care services began their rivalry. Osteopathy had been introduced in 1892 by Dr. Andrew Taylor Still, three years before the discovery of the principles of chiropractic. The success of medical doctors over other health-care services may have come about almost entirely through the increased interest in chemistry. The criticism heaped on osteopathy was also thrust onto chiropractic by the medical or allopathic profession. Apparently, medical doctors tried to monopolize health care.

Practicing health care based on two concepts—physical removal of a diseased area by surgery (considered barbaric by some health-care practitioners) and the use of drugs and narcotics (rooted in antiquity through a long tradition of using herbs)—medical doctors, always in the majority, did not easily accept alternative medical techniques.

Today, chiropractors often use techniques other than pure spinal manipulation. Although chiropractors do not prescribe drugs or practice surgery, in some areas they may use physiotherapy, recommend vitamins and mineral supplements, and (in Nevada) deliver babies. In addition, chiropractors use braces and casts, diathermy machines, whirlpool baths, ultrasound, hot/cold packs, and similar techniques.

CHAPTER II

A Brief Picture
of a Chiropractor's Day

Our typical chiropractor, Dr. C., practices in a small town of about 30,000 people. He has been in practice for twelve years and is well known and liked in the community. His office is in a neighborhood business district a short drive from his home, where he lives with his wife and their two children.

Dr. C.'s office is crowded when he arrives. Ms. B., his nurse, greets him with a smile. She has been with Dr. C. for ten years and enjoys working the four and a half days a week that the office is open.

The first patient to see Dr. C. is Mr. H., a nineteen-year-old who recently was turned down when he tried to enlist in the U.S. Air Force. The examining physician at the recruiting office informed him that he has a spinal curvature that makes him unfit for military duty. He was not aware of this before, although he had noticed that his suits didn't fit well because one shoulder seemed higher than the other. He has been recommended to Dr. C. by his uncle, who has been a patient for many years.

Dr. C. greets Mr. H. cordially and professionally. The chiropractic physician then proceeds to take a detailed case history of the patient. When the history is completed, Dr. C. takes

Mr. H. into another room that contains an X-ray machine, a HI-LO table, a side posture table, and all other necessary diagnostic equipment.

Mr. H. is asked to take his shirt off and the doctor begins to perform tests on the patient. Neurological, orthopedic, and chiropractic examinations are conducted. The doctor takes two 14 x 17-inch X-rays of the lumbar-dorsal area and two 8 x 10-inch X-rays of the cervical area. Mr. H. gets dressed, and the nurse gives him an appointment to return in two days.

The chiropractic physician, in the interim, studies the X-rays and the case history and determines that Mr. H. has a condition called tertiary scoliosis.

When Mr. H. arrives for his next appointment, the doctor takes him into the adjusting room, asks him to remove his shirt and explains the X-rays to him. Mr. H. is told that he has tertiary scoliosis and that treatment requires skillful manipulation of the affected area. He is put on the HI-LO table and moved downward into a stationary position, whereupon Dr. C. makes some adjustments to the affected vertebrae. The patient is then asked to sit up and a neurocalometer is moved up and down his spinal column for a reading.

Mr. H. will begin a program of treatments in the office approximately three times a week. The chiropractor tells him that because his body is still young, a series of adjustments and proper exercise will probably correct the scoliosis without surgery or a back brace.

Naturally, as in any health-care problem, there is no way to guarantee recovery. The doctor can only use the best of his skills. If the patient follows the specified program carefully, he should achieve success.

Dr. C. sees his next patient, Ms. R., who tells him of the ache in her lower back. She has consulted a medical doctor, who prescribed medication and bed rest. The pain has not cleared up.

Dr. C. carefully discusses her problem with her. He examines her spine with his fingertips (a procedure known as *palpation*) and decides that X-rays are not necessary at this point. After positioning her correctly on the HI-LO table, he makes the required adjustment. She says she thinks she is a little better, but she is not sure.

Ms. R. is given some exercise therapy and is requested to make another appointment in a few days. If she is like most patients with lower-back problems, after the next visit to Dr. C. she will notice improvement, and within two weeks the problem will be cleared up.

The third patient, Mr. D., complains of pain in his legs. Many other patients that the chiropractor will see during this day may complain of pains and aches in various parts of their bodies besides the back or spine. Yet there are techniques to help them. The key concept of chiropractic is that subluxations of the spine can cause problems to appear in these other areas. When the spine is correctly adjusted, the pain and discomfort in those areas will stop.

This is not to say that the illness could not be caused by other factors. The modern chiropractor is aware of this, and he uses a variety of methods and techniques and in some cases refers patients to other health-care practitioners.

Almost all chiropractors (86.6 percent of those surveyed by the ACA) own their own X-ray equipment.

The chiropractor's office may also include an Anatomotor or a Spinalator—automated tables that may combine massage, traction, heat, and vibration.

According to a study conducted by Dr. R. C. Shafer of the ACA, 83.3 percent of the physicians used one or more physiotherapeutic procedures such as ultrasound, traction, sinewave, diathermy, infrared, ultraviolet, pulsed diathermy, percussion, mechanotherapy, cryogenics, hydrotherapy, colotherapy, oxygen inhalation, and paraffin therapy.

How does the treatment of patients by a chiropractor differ

from the treatment given by a medical doctor or an osteopath? Chiropractic is built upon three related scientific principles. The first is that disease can be caused by disturbances of the nervous system. There may be many other factors that cause poor health, but the introduction of agents and conditions that irritate the central nervous system can cause deviation from the norm.

Second, disturbances of the nervous system may be caused by derangements of the musculoskeletal structure. Strains and stresses within the musculoskeletal system caused by man's erect posture may cause subluxation—a mechanical, chemical, or psychic irritation of the nervous system.

Third, disturbances of the nervous system may cause or aggravate disease in various parts or functions of the body. Subluxation may trigger or start headaches and other types of aches and pains through reactions with other bodily components.

In order to treat the patient, the chiropractor follows a specific set of procedures. First, he interviews the patient and develops a profile. Second, he conducts a thorough and systematic physical examination using standard methods, techniques, and instruments. He conducts a postural and spinal analysis. Third, he uses diagnostic aids—particularly the X-ray. Finally, he conducts laboratory tests, which can include cytology, hematology, bacteriology, and parasitology.

Next, the chiropractor uses treatment methods that do not include prescription drugs or surgery. Instead, he attempts to correct the subluxation by means of adjusting the vertebrae by a physical thrust.

In addition, the modern chiropractor may also supervise the patient's dietary and nutritional needs to avoid dysfunctions. He may use or suggest physiotherapeutic measures such as exercise and give other professional counsel in posture or sanitation.

Although the central purpose of chiropractic is to treat the whole person, the scope of chiropractic practice is described specifically by law, which sometimes varies from state to state.

Further, some chiropractors believe in adapting certain techniques whereas others do not. Traditionally, the two schools have been called "straights" and "mixers." The "straights" use only spinal adjustments for treatment of all disease; the "mixers" borrow and adapt freely from the other health professions.

CHAPTER III

What Personal Qualities Make a Good Chiropractor?

You should possess certain personal qualities if you are to become a good student and a successful practitioner of chiropractic. No one of these characteristics is more important than any other, yet you need them all.

You must enjoy learning. Further, you should like thinking and studying, because you must be a good student with a good amount of intelligence to succeed in chiropractic college. As a practitioner, you will need to spend the rest of your life studying the science and skill of your craft.

Specifically, *you must excel in science.* Your years of training will be based on an understanding of very fundamental and basic scientific concepts that you are expected to have mastered by the time you gain admittance to the college of chiropractic.

You must like people. Although you need not be the life of the party, you should be able to get along with almost everyone. As a practitioner of the healing arts you can expect to treat people of every race, color, and creed, and from every level of society. Further, you must be compassionate, considerate, and sympathetic. You will be seeing people at their worst, when they are in pain or otherwise distraught and in many cases not acting pleasantly. They will come to you to help them.

You should be emotionally stable to deal with crises that will occur during your college training and in overcharged emotional situations like the ones you will encounter with your patients. Not everyone can maintain a cool head in a crisis, and that is what will often be expected of you. The manner you develop must be calm and self-assured to help you help your patient and to keep him from becoming further upset.

You must be willing to accept responsibility. Many people are unwilling to do this, although they may be willing and able to do something if they are told what to do. Not only must you take action, but you must be sure that you know what you are doing and accept responsibility for it.

You must be able to adapt and adjust to a wide range of circumstances. Even though your training will teach you what to do, each human is different and you will have to be ingenious and intelligent enough to see what will work with certain patients and what will not. Failures are a part of life, and you'll have to expect some; however, your goal must be to keep your failures to a minimum and not to let them overwhelm and defeat you.

You must be able to organize your activities. If you can't get yourself started, you would find it difficult to be a chiropractor. There is a demand for organization, from planning your day, to ordering and maintaining your equipment and supplies, to billing your patients and keeping records. It is true that after you are established, you can get an assistant to do much of that, but you will have to understand what needs to be done. Further, without a sense of organization and purpose you will not be able to give the best possible health care to your patients. The ability to plan and carry out your work is extremely important to your success as a professional.

You must have a respect for the profession. Even though the monetary rewards are high, chiropractic is not a profession one should enter for the financial benefits alone. There is a great amount of prestige and respect in and for the profession that should be maintained. Thus, a sense of ethics and moral duty is a prime prerequisite of the person who wishes to enter this field. It is a profession with room only for those of the highest moral character. Your major goal, therefore, should be the ethical and honest discharge of your professional duties to your patients.

Physical Dexterity in Chiropractic

To be a successful chiropractic physician, you need to be in good health and to possess sufficient qualities of endurance to reach your goal of helping your patients. However, you do not have to be exceptionally strong physically. The key is agility with your hands. It would be difficult for anyone lacking the full use of his extremities to give the patients the full manipulations needed for corrective adjustments.

Of course, it is obvious that good natural or corrected eyesight and hearing are important. Other than these obvious things, normal good health should be a necessary consideration of anyone who wishes to enter any of the healing arts.

Why an Interest in Natural Living Is a Good Beginning

Although natural foods are often thought of as a fad (and rightly so, in some instances), there is much to be said in favor of diets that do not contain foods with a high amount of artificial ingredients. Over the years since the creation of the Pure Food Laws in 1895, the government has been trying to control what processors put into food. They have not been entirely successful.

Every day we read about red dye, DES, and similar substances that the government has found to be dangerous but that are being put into food. If you are aware of these dangerous substances, you can avoid foods containing them.

Chiropractic goes a step beyond simply demanding that the body be protected from these unnatural and often harmful chemicals (whose purpose often is only to keep the food from spoiling during long storage). The art and science of chiropractic believes that the human body will heal itself. It is necessary to keep the body attuned to the natural balance provided by nature.

Thus, if you are interested in natural processes of living, the philosophy of chiropractic should be very appealing.

CHAPTER IV

How to Prepare for Chiropractic College

If you are still in high school when you begin planning your chiropractic career, you will be able to take specific courses that will be of great help to your success. For example, your high-school curriculum should include as many science courses as possible. Take chemistry, biology, and any other courses that are offered in those areas. Your guidance counselor can help you plan your schedule.

If, like many people, you are a high-school graduate seeking a career in the healing arts, you can enroll in a community college or a four-year college with a prechiropractic major (or if that is not offered, an allied-health major or a premed major). If you are not a high-school graduate, it is possible to obtain a high-school equivalency diploma, which may make you eligible to attend college for prechiropractic training. Check with your local high school for further information.

A recommended prechiropractic college curriculum would include the following courses:

First Year—First Semester	*Credits*
Freshman English	3
General Chemistry	5

First Year—First Semester	*Credits*
General Zoology	4
College Algebra	3
Physical Education	1
	16

First Year—Second Semester	*Credits*
Freshman English	3
General Chemistry	5
Anatomy and Physiology	5
Fundamentals of Speech	2
Physical Education	1
	16

Second Year—First Semester	*Credits*
General Physics	4
Organic Chemistry	4
General Psychology	3
American Government	3
Principles of Economics	3
	17

Second Year—Second Semester	*Credits*
General Physics	4
Organic Chemistry	4
Abnormal Psychology	3
General Bacteriology	4
Introduction to Sociology	3
	18

Remember that successful completion of these courses is the minimum entrance requirement of most chiropractic colleges. Recently, many colleges of chiropractic have been stiffening admission requirements by increasing the number of credits in biology and chemistry as prerequisites.

You will also notice that there is an emphasis on the prospective chiropractor's getting a liberal education as well as a scientific one. In keeping with the idea of the interdependence of mind and body and of maintaining the ecological balance of all the facets of man, chiropractic science insists that its practitioners should not be narrow in their education but be intelligent people with a broad spectrum of knowledge.

Even though a student may gain admission to many chiropractic colleges with a minimum of two years' preparation (which could be obtained in many good community colleges), he may do better with an even more advanced educational preparation such as three or four years. In fact, about 45 percent of the students now entering chiropractic college have a B.A. or a B.S. degree. Many practitioners believe that in the near future a bachelor's degree will be the minimum requirement for entrance into an accredited college of chiropractic.

All states have specific educational requirements for the chiropractor. Minimum standards set by these states range from a high-school equivalency diploma (plus a degree from an accredited college of chiropractic) in Alabama, to two years of college or university training (required by most states). In actual practice, however, it is unlikely that anyone with only a high-school equivalency diploma could gain admittance to chiropractic college or be able to keep up with the requirements of the conventional curriculum unless he had successfully completed two years or more of prechiropractic college training.

As part of the steadily increasing upgrading of standards of chiropractic colleges, most require a minimum of one college-level course in biology and one in chemistry for entrance. Although you may find it possible to gain admittance with a C average, your chance will improve if your grade average is higher. In the past five years, it has become increasingly difficult to gain admittance.

CHAPTER V

Planning Your College Career

If you are like most students of chiropractic, you'll enter chiropractic college at 24.4 years of age after having worked for one year after high school and after having attended a college or university for two and a half years.

Most likely you will have been a chiropractic patient and have received information about the profession from your chiropractic physician.

The chiropractic profession is quite concerned that its new members receive a good education. In 1947 the American Chiropractic Association, then called the National Chiropractic Association, formed the Council of Chiropractic Education (CCE) to upgrade professional education. Colleges accredited by the CCE are required to be nonprofit institutions employing faculty members who have a graduate degree and clinical experience in their field. The college must have adequate laboratory facilities and a clinic.

Since October 1, 1980, forty-eight states have agreed that all applicants for licenses must have graduated from a chiropractic college accredited by the CCE or the equivalent.

Presently, nine schools are fully accredited and have a total enrollment of 9,267 students. They are:

Los Angeles College of Chiropractic, Glendale, California
National College of Chiropractic, Lombard, Illinois
Northwestern College of Chiropractic, St. Paul, Minnesota
Texas Chiropractic College, Pasadena, Texas
Cleveland Chiropractic College, Kansas City, Missouri
Logan College of Chiropractic, Chesterfield, Missouri
New York Chiropractic College, Glen Head, New York
Palmer College of Chiropractic, Davenport, Iowa
Western States Chiropractic College, Portland, Oregon

Choosing a College

There are several decisions to make in choosing a college. The first is location. Usually you should choose a nearby college because it will reduce your expenses; you don't need to pay for relocating in an area that you might not like. The only alternative is to attempt to choose a college in a low-cost area if it is possible for you to move there.

Another decision is to determine whether you wish to attend an accredited or an unaccredited college. Simply stated, an accredited college is one whose courses, faculty, and facilities have been examined and judged adequate by a board of examiners. Unaccredited colleges usually are new institutions that have not been in operation long enough to be considered or examined by the board.

The courses of study and the instruction may be excellent in an unaccredited college. However, you do run the risk that the school, for some reason, may not be accepted for accreditation and that your degree would be worthless. This happens, but colleges usually prepare carefully so that they meet all the requirements. The advantages of attending an unaccredited college are that it is usually easier to gain admittance and there is the thrill and excitement of being part of a new institution.

Even though most students attend chiropractic colleges in the United States, you are free to apply to a foreign college. Many are located in English-speaking countries, and thus there is no language barrier. However, travel expenses and the lack of fellowships and scholarships may be hindrances. After graduation, you still must take and pass the National Board examinations. The attrition or dropout rate is low—far less than the 20 percent expected in medical colleges.

College officials will weigh your application against a number of factors—your grades in high school and in your two years of prechiropractic training, your extracurricular activities (sports, debating teams, and other activities that offer evidence of your ability to adapt and get along with others).

International students must meet the same preprofessional academic criteria as American students. Further, international students must have valid documents of admission to the United States. If any questions arise about the American equivalency of the student's international training, it is the responsibility of the student to obtain a letter of explanation and approval from the CCE.

Students can obtain *advanced standing* in some cases. You need to check carefully with your chosen college for its rules and regulations. Usually students requesting advanced standing are required to prove that the courses they have completed are equivalent to those of the college. If the school from which the student wishes to transfer credits is not accredited by the CCE, the courses are accepted only on a provisional basis. Advanced standing for courses taken at an accredited liberal-arts college are often granted for hours above the 60-semester-hour prerequisite.

How to Handle the Personal Interview

Since you are in competition for a seat in the entering class, you can expect a personal interview even if your grades are high and you have the best references. Often the interviewer will do everything he can to put you at ease, although this is not always the case.

You can think about some of the questions that the interviewer might ask you and outline what you might say. Usually the questions will run something like this: Why do you want to be a chiropractor? How much contact have you had with chiropractic? What do you know about the field? Are you interested in science? Do you make friends easily?

Put yourself at ease and answer the questions as honestly as you can. Don't attempt to put on a false front. Try to keep your answers short and clear; don't ramble. Try to direct your answer to the reason the question is relevant to your future career.

If you are really concerned about the interview, use the technique of role-playing. Have one of your friends query you with typical questions. Seek the advice of a guidance counselor. Most important, visit your chiropractor and ask his advice, for it will be the most worthwhile of all.

Ways to Make the College Want to Admit You

Show the interviewer that you have a sincere interest in chiropractic by your activities. In addition to presenting evidence that you are active in your community (which shows interest in helping others), join chiropractic organizations available to you.

CHAPTER VI

How Much Will It Cost?

The only sure thing about your expenses is that they will always be higher than you think. Make an estimate, but be sure to understand that there will always be unexpected items that will ruin the best-planned budget.

Tuition and Other Expenses and How to Estimate Them

In general, you can expect your tuition to be approximately $1,000 to $1,500 a quarter (or four times that amount if you go year-round).

Most colleges will refund at least part of your tuition if you find it necessary to withdraw before a specified date, which varies from one school to another.

You are required to pay a nonrefundable application fee (usually $25 to $50), a general fee for college activities (often $25), and laboratory fees for many classes (usually $20). These fees are payable by a specified date—usually on enrollment.

In addition, you will have to purchase books and other supplies, which can range from $150 to $500 or more a semester.

Of course, living expenses are in addition to these expenses. Few colleges of chiropractic have dormitories or apartments available to students. To live in the city is more expensive than living in the country, so it is difficult to give a precise estimate of living expenses. Obviously it will cost just about what it costs you now.

You will be required to purchase equipment and supplies such as the following:

Physician's bag
Chiropractic Speeder
Thermocouple Instrument
Stethoscope
Sphygmomanometer (aneroid or mercurial)
Otoscope
Ophthalmoscope (Fibre Optic Lens System)
Oral Thermometer with case
Rectal Thermometer with case
Neurological Hammer (having a pin and brush)
Tuning Forks Weighted Heads (256cc and 128cc)
Linen tape measure
Tongue depressors
Whartenberg Wheel
Red and black skin-marking pencils
Pocket flashlight
Pry Rule for Logan Basic Methods
Gonstead Equipment and Notes
Grostoc Equipment and Notes
Sections of the Human Spine, Vertebrae Articulations
Dissection Kit

It is usually not necessary to purchase a microscope, since one will be provided for your use. Prices are not listed for the items in the diagnostic kit because they are subject to change. You can expect to pay about $400 for these materials.

In summary, then, a chiropractic education in an accredited

chiropractic college costs about the same as training in medicine or osteopathy.

More complete information about costs can be found by consulting current chiropractic college catalogs or by writing to individual colleges or state and national chiropractic professional organizations.

How to Obtain Financial Aid

Financial aid in the form of scholarships and loans is available to you from a variety of sources: local, regional, and national. Generally, you apply through the Financial Aid Office of the college.

On a *local* level, you will find some funds available from alumni bequests made to the chiropractic college in which you are enrolled. Criteria for granting these scholarships usually have one or more stipulations to make the selection of recipients easier. For example, in a typical college a grant of $500 may be made annually to a student from California (students from other states are ineligible), or $25 per quarter will be paid by a sponsoring doctor and matched by the college for a total of $50 to any applicant maintaining a 3.5 average or better. Sometimes short-term loans are made on similar bases.

In addition, on a *regional* level, there are both private and state-funded scholarships and grants ranging from $25 to $500 and more. Loans are sometimes available as well. Usually there are stipulations that the recipient live in a particular area or meet some other specific requirement.

National scholarships and loans are also available. Students enrolled in certified chiropractic colleges are eligible for guaranteed student loans, National Defense Student Loans, student work-study programs, and Interest Assistance Programs. They may also qualify for vocational-rehabilitation tuition and maintenance programs. The Veterans Administration recognizes chiropractic colleges as institutions of higher learning, and veterans may utilize benefits obtainable under the G.I. Bill.

Short-term emergency loans for chiropractic students are made by a national organization, the Reginald Gold Loan Fund, which was established by the Patient Association for Chiropractic Education (PACE). These loans must be repaid no later than three years after graduation.

Obtain specific information about financial aid available from your selected chiropractic college.

Alternative Ways of Financing Your Chiropractic Education

Most colleges have a *deferred tuition plan* that permits paying tuition in three equal installments. Usually there is a small service charge of less than $10 a semester. In some cases it is cheaper to borrow the entire amount at bank rates, pay for your tuition, and then repay the loan before the end of the semester.

There are often work opportunities near chiropractic colleges. However, you will be limited in the number of hours that you will be available for work because you will need to spend many hours in class and in study. Further, your earnings will be low because most jobs offering the flexible hours that you need will be for temporary and unskilled workers. If at all possible, you should not work while you are attending chiropractic college, because you will need to put your entire energies into learning your profession.

CHAPTER VII

What Will You Study?

Your chiropractic education will have two major divisions: basic scientific subjects and clinical subjects. Your time will be divided roughly between them, with slightly more time spent in the clinical area in many schools.

In the first year in a college of chiropractic you will study the subjects that will be the foundation of your profession. These basic sciences are the same ones that are studied in colleges of medicine, although the approach is different. Your courses will be taught by professors trained in the specialties of psychology, anatomy, chemistry, physiology, pathology, and roentgenology.

You will study the philosophy and history of chiropractic, so that you will understand the nature and development of your profession. The basics of spinal mechanics and various adjusting techniques (spinology) will be covered extensively. In addition, you will study embryology (analysis of the cell, chromosomes, genetic factors, and hereditary diseases) and histology (including the preparation, pathology, and analysis of tissues).

Further classes in your first year will introduce you to the techniques, theories, and procedures of using X-rays (roentgenology), inorganic chemistry, pathology, and similar subjects. Great emphasis is placed on anatomy, both in theory and in lab sessions where you engage in dissection of higher primates under careful supervision.

In short, your studies will not only introduce you to the theories and philosophies of chiropractic but will also start you on your way through the intense study of complex chemical and skeletomuscular subjects so that you gain a basic understanding of them. The first year is vitally important, for here you will gain the basics that you need for an understanding of more complicated concepts. In addition, you will see the practical application of what you are learning.

The second year will continue your study of the basic areas with organic chemistry, microbiology, anatomy, pathology, and similar subjects that students in all of the healing-arts professions study. In addition, however, you will begin to see how chiropractic principles are embedded in some of these major concepts.

There will be various courses in technic, proceeding from a basic cervical pressure technic on to more involved procedures. You will receive clinical instruction and learn laboratory and physical diagnosis techniques and procedures. You will spend a lot of time studying advanced X-ray physics and placement.

By this time you will be becoming quite knowledgeable in the basics of your profession. You will be approaching the halfway point at which the completion of your training is within sight and you can work toward the last two years of your program.

Your third year will cover biochemistry (which includes carbohydrates, proteins, enzymes, and similar items) as well as pediatrics and obstetrics. In addition, you will work with patients (under supervision in the clinic). Public health is an important part of your program as well.

In your fourth year, you will continue with laboratory diagnosis, pathology, gynecology, and toxicology. You will spend many hours in the clinic. You will spend time in lectures, demonstrations, and in actual participation in treatment in the clinic, taking case histories, performing physical examinations, and studying the physical conditions of patients under the supervision of a clinical director.

Although we have gone over them in a very general way, in your four years you will have spent in class approximately 880 hours in anatomy, 352 hours in chemistry, 480 hours in diagnosis, 208 hours in microbiology, 304 hours in pathology, 320 hours in physiology, 176 hours in public health and first aid, 272 hours in roentgenology, 64 hours in on-departmental required courses (like psychology), 1,200 hours in chiropractic and related courses, 904 hours in clinical instruction and the required externship, for a grand total of 5,160 hours (although this may vary slightly from college to college). The C.E.E. stipulates a standard basic curriculum.

Most colleges of chiropractic have clinics for their undergraduates in which the student observes, records his findings, and discusses the patient's progress. These records are then discussed and evaluated by his clinical supervisor. Further, he begins to work with classmates in spinal adjustments on patients in the clinic, again under supervision. (This is sometimes called an externship.)

Graduate clinics are also an important part of continuing the education process. Clinical patients and patients with special problems are examined and adjustments are made with special study groups under supervision by a faculty member.

Of course, college life is not all study. Chiropractic colleges like other institutions of higher learning have class organizations, fraternities and sororities, publications (including the college newspaper and yearbook), student councils, and community involvement in many activities. You will find lots to keep you busy!

CHAPTER VIII

Getting Your License

What Your License Means

As a means of safeguarding the public from poor health care, strict licensing regulations have been established for practitioners of all the healing arts.

After completing your two years of preprofessional training, and after graduation from an accredited college with the degree of Doctor of Chiropractic, you are required to pass an examination in the state in which you intend to practice.

Requirements vary from state to state. In some states, you first must pass separate examinations in chemistry, physiology, anatomy, microbiology, pathology, and public health before you can apply for licensing.

Further, in some states the examining board is composed entirely of Doctors of Chiropractic; in others, medical doctors comprise all or part of the licensing board, which in this case is called a "Mixed Board."

Although all fifty states have license requirements, passing the examination in one state does not permit you to practice in another.

The National Board of Chiropractor Examiners has developed

a chiropractic examination program for use at the national level that provides a service for state boards of examiners, chiropractic colleges, and the graduate chiropractor.

A student is eligible to take the exam when certified by the dean or registrar of his college. If you wait more than eight months after graduation to apply for the test, you must furnish a letter from your state society or from the secretary of the board of examiners in the state in which you practice or have practiced.

The National Boards are now administered twice a year. There are two parts.

Part One consists of the following:

Anatomy
1. General
2. Spinal
Physiology
Chemistry
Pathology
Microbiology—hygiene, sanitation

Part Two consists of the following:

Diagnosis
1. Physical, clinical, laboratory
2. Chiropractic-oriented diagnosis (neuromusculoskeletal)
X-ray
Principles and Practices
1. Principles
2. Associated Clinical Sciences
   Gynecology, obstetrics, pediatrics, geriatrics, dermatology, syphilology, toxicology, psychology, psychiatry, jurisprudence, ethics, economics
Physiotherapy (parachiropractic therapeutics)

Each exam covers a three-day period instead of the previous four. All thirteen subjects are administered with a testing period of one and a half hours for each subject and a fifteen-minute break. The present number of test sites is twelve—ten in the United States, one in England, and one in Canada.

There is a National Board policy that no more than two subjects in a part can be retaken—except the physiotherapy elective. There is an extra charge for this.

Applications may be obtained from the office of the dean of any chiropractic college or by writing to National Board of Chiropractic Examiners, 1610 Twenty-ninth Avenue Place, Greeley, Colorado 80631.

The fee for examination in most states varies from $100 to $150. At present, most state examining boards accept the examination from the National Board of Chiropractic Examiners. In addition, there is usually a day-long clinical examination that the applicant must pass. Once the license is obtained, it is usually good for two years. Renewal is automatic; the Doctor of Chiropractic need only fill out a form answering such questions as have to do with his maintaining good moral character and ethical conduct.

Once the license is obtained, it becomes a precious possession for the doctor, for he must exercise wisdom, integrity, and intelligence throughout his career to maintain the license.

The following is a current list of states that recognize the National Board of Chiropractic Examiners:

STATE CHIROPRACTIC BOARDS
(and Mixed Boards that License Chiropractors)

Alabama	Delaware	Illinois
Alaska	District of Columbia	Indiana
Arizona	Florida	Iowa
Arkansas	Georgia	Kansas
California	Hawaii	Kentucky
Colorado	Idaho	Louisiana

Maine
Maryland
Massachusetts
Michigan
Minnesota
Mississippi
Missouri
Montana
Nebraska
Nevada
New Hampshire

New Jersey
New Mexico
New York
North Carolina
North Dakota
Oklahoma
Ohio
Oregon
Pennsylvania
Rhode Island
South Dakota

Tennessee'
Texas
Utah
Vermont
Virginia
Washington
West Virginia
Wyoming

CHAPTER IX

Setting Up Your Practice

So the day has finally arrived! You've graduated from chiropractic college as a Doctor of Chiropractic. You've passed the state boards, you've received your license, and you are ready to set up practice. You are now confronted by several alternatives. You can set up a new office, purchase an established practice, or join together with a partner or a chiropractic group.

Of course, you could choose one of the alternative careers mentioned in Chapter X. You alone make the decision.

What do you need to do in setting up a new office? It is unethical for a chiropractic physician to advertise in a flambuoyant or misleading manner. He may put a small notice in the newspapers announcing that he is opening an office. Of course, he may list his name under Chiropractors in the Yellow Pages of the telephone directory.

Chiropractors' patients spread the word. You'll have a dignified sign outside your office. This is also limited in most states. You are permitted to have only your name and D.C. or Chiropractic Physician after it. As time goes by, patients will start coming in.

In addition, you may find that a local factory or other business will refer employees to you. Chiropractic care is now covered under many insurance plans.

Besides getting patients, you will need to get equipment that you have learned to use while earning your degree. Every chiropractic office needs chairs and tables for the patients' waiting room. That often goes with the office.

Equipment such as an X-ray machine and the neurocalometer, adjustment tables, and similar items can run close to $25,000 or $50,000. Because of this enormous expense, some firms will arrange with the new chiropractor to purchase all the equipment and then lease it or let him pay in installments over many years.

A chiropractor can incorporate his practice to gain certain legal and tax advantages, although fewer than one out of ten do so.

You can, of course, purchase an established practice. For example, you'll find ads in *The ACA Journal of Chiropractic* offering a fully established practice for sale, including a furnished office and equipment. This has advantages and disadvantages.

The advantages are that you won't have to wait long to start receiving a steady flow of patients. You won't have to struggle along making do without specific pieces of equipment that you need.

On the other hand, you may find that since the physician is retiring, much of his equipment is old—he purchased it when he first set up his practice thirty years ago. In addition, there is no assurance that you will continue to see the same patients he sees; they may decide to go elsewhere when they hear that he is retiring. Finally, you may find the whole thing far too expensive and impossible for you to finance successfully.

You may decide to go into practice with an already established physician, using his office and equipment and seeing some of his patients. Or you may decide to make an arrangement that will permit you to use another professional's office during hours when he isn't there. There are various alternatives to starting a new office, but that is what many chiropractors must do. For example, in many sections of the country there is no established practice for you to take over even if you wanted to. Because of the severe shortage of chiropractic physicians, most of them are centralized in cities. If you want a country or small-town practice, you will almost always have to set it up new.

If you set up a partnership, you agree to share expenses and income with another chiropractic physician. Obviously, this arrangement works well only in a city large enough to provide a sufficient number of patients for both of you. You may decide that you wish to join a chiropractic group. This arrangement is popular because practitioners of the chiropractic art can group together in one building with adequate parking and a shared receptionist and in this manner cut down on overhead.

CHAPTER X

Careers Other Than Private Practice

Most doctors of chiropractic are self-employed. They have established a private practice, which in the average week permits them to attend to the needs of one hundred or more patients. However, some chiropractic physicians do not like private practice for a variety of reasons, such as the long hours that are sometimes required, or the financial risk that needs to be taken for several years while the practice is being built up.

Thus, some chiropractors are employed by other chiropractors, are employed by industry, practice in a clinic or large hospital such as Spears, or are engaged in research or teaching. Of these, the most common alternatives are *teaching* and *research*.

Teaching chiropractic offers great personal rewards. It is a way in which you can influence an enormous number of people. By imparting your knowledge and skills to your students, you will be doing them a service. Don't overlook the fact, however, that your students will teach their knowledge to their patients and they (and perhaps even their patients) may become teachers of chiropractic, too, thus passing along the wisdom of scholars, researchers, and practitioners in this health field.

Most chiropractic physicians who teach have a practice as well, even though they may be limited in the amount of time and effort they can devote to it. And, of course, by working with patients at the college at which they teach, and keeping up with the latest techniques in the field, their knowledge of chiropractic grows.

In fact, it would be fatal if a chiropractor stopped learning after he received his degree. As with any of the healing arts, new discoveries are being made all the time. Thus he needs to keep up with them so that he can give his patients the best possible help. There are ample opportunities for chiropractors to present papers at national conventions or to teach graduate seminars, thereby imparting a knowledge of their specialty to their fellow physicians.

Research is also interesting. Like the other health professions, chiropractic encourages its practitioners to engage in research. It is, in fact, very dependent upon studies made in the basic sciences. Modern chiropractors acknowledge that too often in the past practitioners have looked upon it mainly as an applied science.

Although millions of dollars are poured into medical research projects by the federal government, chiropractic researchers have not received this support. Recently this has been changing. The Department of Health, Education, and Welfare and the Department of Labor appropriation bill recently allocated $2 million for chiropractic research, which is included in the budgets of the National Institute of Neurological Diseases and Strokes (NINDS) and the National Institutes of Health (NIH).

For example, The National College of Chiropractic received a grant of $24,969 to examine certain standards in the measurement of X-ray levels.

Most completed research has been done with the use of private funds and through the Foundation of Chiropractic Education and Research, where 12 percent of the ACA education budget is allocated to research. As more government funds become available, research in chiropractic will increase enormously, and both the practitioner and the patient will benefit.

Research appeals to many practitioners. Although they enjoy working with people and helping them to get well, they find it more fascinating to work on the very frontiers of their science, exploring promising new avenues of health care.

You, too, might enjoy, for example, finding new ways to make corrective adjustments while using the same established techniques that chiropractic physicians have used for years. You might be interested in gathering statistical data showing the chances of recovery from certain conditions through the use of chiropractic care.

Practicing chiropractic physicians also do research. You can see the results of their studies in such prestigious publications as *The ACA Journal of Chiropractic*. For instance, in a recent issue, Dr. A. C. Larcher contributed an important article on football injuries, which analyzes traumatic myositis ossificans (formation of calcium in unusual amounts one half inch wide and four or five inches long), a condition that is painful and may require surgery. He details methods found successful in treating it.

In another article, Dr. Andrew R. Jessen discusses whether intervertebral discs are shock absorbers or shock transmitters, and what this means to the practice of chiropractic.

Further intraprofessional studies have been carried out on projects such as the following:

1. Neutron radiography of connective tissues and other soft tissues.
2. Use of cineradiography and static films to correlate the dynamics of spinal and pelvic movements.
3. Obtaining of data regarding possible relative movement between sacrum and innominate bones.
4. Investigation by a qualified physicist concerning the valid-

ity of measurements obtained through chiropractic diagnostic instruments.

Studies of this nature move the art and science of chiropractic health care forward. Just as research is extensive in the other medical sciences, chiropractors develop new methods, processes, and ideas through the meticulous study of their craft.

CHAPTER XI

What You Can Expect to Earn

When your practice is established, your earnings in the profession of chiropractic will have no limits. It is true that at the beginning your income will be low; but that is because it will take some time to build up a practice. Meanwhile, you may also engage in other professional work such as practicing part-time in a chiropractic hospital or clinic. Soon, however, if you put to use conscientiously what you've been taught, your practice will begin to snowball and you'll have more patients than you can handle.

Your Income and How It Will Grow

Apparently few people become chiropractors because of a desire for prestige and a higher income. One research study found that almost half of the students surveyed (42 percent) chose the profession because they had personally benefited from chiropractic. About one quarter (24 percent) believed in natural healing methods; 15 percent of the students had a desire to help others, and only 3 percent chose chiropractic because of the financial rewards that it offered.

Even though you enter the healing-arts profession to contribute to human betterment and not just for the money, as a chiropractor you are assured of earning an income beyond the average. According to the American Chiropractic Association, after ten years the typical Doctor of Chiropractic treats one hundred patients or more in his usual four-and-a-half-day week, and thus his income is on the same level as that of other health-care professionals.

According to the ACA, the typical chiropractor's income (after paying office expenses) ranges upward of $40,000. Obviously this depends on many factors such as location, economic conditions, and the ability of the chiropractic physician.

In addition, like other health-care professionals, the Doctor of Chiropractic enjoys security and prestige. As your practice continues, it will expand. Since it is unethical to advertise, it will grow through your patients' recommendations to their friends and acquaintances.

Your opportunities are enormous. You may wish to expand into larger offices or establish a clinic or hospital. There is no limit to your income or challenge. Your chosen profession will be an honorable career, helpful to mankind, and offering services to those who need it. For this you will be well rewarded financially, but even more important, you will also receive the respect of your patients and the community.

It will take you a few years to become established. If you decide to set up practice in a small town or a rural area, it may take a shorter time; in a large city, it may take slightly longer. In all the healing-arts professions, physicians practicing in small towns usually make more money than those practicing in large cities.

Part of building your practice will be to educate your patients as to what chiropractic is and what it can do for them. In cities where chiropractic has been established, this may be less of a problem than in some small towns or rural areas.

Most chiropractors are self-employed. In addition to their

practice they may teach at a chiropractic college or they may be affiliated with a large chiropractic hospital or clinic. Unlike other health-care professionals, chiropractors usually do not find salaried full-time positions outside of private practice. They also do not find opportunities of offering their health-care service in the armed service.

But they can find security in their own practices. Blue Shield, Medicaid, health and accident insurance, and welfare pay the chiropractic physician directly. Since most of his payments come from these sources, he is assured of receiving payment and thus has security. In addition, some chiropractic physicians maintain contracts with industry to treat members of unions and other groups an unlimited number of times for a set yearly fee.

Personal Satisfactions from Your Work

Perhaps even more important than the financial rewards of your profession will be the enormous satisfaction you will find in helping people.

Chiropractic practitioners find immense satisfaction in seeing the results of their work. People can earn large sums of money on many jobs, yet find them dull and tedious. This is not so in a profession where you will always be challenged.

As you grow older you find out how important your life's work is to you. In scientific research into the attitudes of factory workers, it was found that when they sabotaged their products or destroyed their factories, it was often because they hated their jobs. Mankind seems to need purpose in what he does for a living. Professions are tasks that supply the answer to that need. Chiropractic is a profession that gives purpose to your life.

Further, becoming a chiropractic physician carries with it a great deal of prestige in your community. You are set off from the average person simply because you are a doctor. With that privilege, however, comes a great responsibility. People will expect certain behavior from you and from your family; you will find that they look up to you as a community leader.

It is factors like these that are intangible rewards; they can't be measured in dollars and cents.

CHAPTER XII

Postgraduate Training

You will need to keep up with the expanding knowledge in your field after you graduate from college. Research develops new ideas and new ways of doing things that you will need to know about.

The Need for Constant Learning

Both The American Chiropractic Association and The International Chiropractic Association hold annual conventions that you will want to attend. There are seminars on the science, the art, and the practice of chiropractic that will keep you up to date. For example, at a recent ACA convention there were seminars on such diverse topics as "Practical Aspects of Roentgenolic Quality Control" and "Examination of the Spinal Subluxation Complex by Orthopedic and Neurologic Testing Procedures." Such knowledge will help you in your practice.

You will also keep up with advances in the field by reading professional publications such as *The ACA Journal of Chiropractic*. As you become more skilled in your field you should do some research on your own, with the hope of eventually presenting a paper on it at a national convention or publishing it in a professional journal.

After graduation, you can attend classes at many colleges for a short period to obtain a Bachelor of Arts degree, although about 50 percent of the students now entering chiropractic college already have a B.A. According to a spokesman for the ICA, about 85 percent of the students graduating with a Doctor of Chiropractic degree also elect to fulfill the liberal-arts requirements for a B.A. degree.

Many chiropractors continue their liberal education and earn a Master of Arts degree in a field of their choice, often closely allied to their scientific interests. Others continue toward a Ph.D. (Doctor of Philosophy) or an Ed.D. (Doctor of Education), thus qualifying for a wide range of responsibilities such as teaching or holding an administrative post in a college or university.

The Place of Philosophy in Chiropractic

It may seem in your first two years of training that chiropractic is all memorization, because most of your time then will be spent in learning the names of bones, muscles, and similar technical matters. As time goes on, however, you'll begin to see that chiropractic is not only a knowledge of how things work—the kind of knowledge that a mechanic would have—but that it goes beyond to "why," which is the kind of knowledge of the subject that a philosopher would have.

Although it is not offered at the present time, graduate chiropractors used to work toward a Ph.C. or Philosopher of Chiropractic degree. In this period of study chiropractors discussed and examined what chiropractic is and what it means. Some chiropractors currently think that an advanced degree of some sort, perhaps a Ph.D., will be offered in the next five or ten years —perhaps just in time for you to take it.

The first Ph.D. in Chiropractic Research ever granted was awarded to Dr. S. W. Hsu in 1976 by the University of Colorado. Dr. Hsu's dissertation was a computer analysis of spinal motion as seen by cineroentgenology (X-ray movies). His work may be typical of the postgraduate chiropractic studies of the future.

Even if you never move toward any degree in addition to your D.C. (Doctor of Chiropractic), you will sooner or later have to come to an understanding of what chiropractic is and/or should be. You will have to speculate on man's place in the universe. The basic premise of chiropractic is that there is a certain ecology that man should revere, and that by keeping the balance intact he can improve his health and life. Understanding how this works is part of the study of philosophy in chiropractic.

Refresher Courses and Why They Are Necessary

As research continues and new discoveries are made, you will find that it is hard to keep up with them. In some of the sciences a person's knowledge becomes outdated at a fantastic rate. Five years after a person graduates with a degree in space engineering, everything that he has learned will be changed! Although such startling and rapid changes are not guaranteed to happen in chiropractic, you can be sure that some changes will occur.

Obviously, you must be prepared for them. If you are like most people in the healing arts, you'll enjoy keeping up with what is new as a means of improving your skill and helping your patients.

You can do this by reading the journals, of course, and by attending seminars at conventions. One major problem that the chiropractor faces is that he practices alone, unlike members of the other healing-arts professions who practice at hospitals and thus receive new ideas presented by their fellow practitioners.

Thus, you are sure to find that postgraduate courses are a vital part of your professional career. As an example, the National Lincoln School of Postgraduate Education, which is a division of the National College of Chiropractic, offers a typical postgraduate course on weekends (so that you do not miss valuable office time) in Practical Chiropractic Radiology. Five twelve-hour segments deal with highly advanced radiological techniques. Other courses similar to this offered by accredited institutions are invaluable.

CHAPTER XIII

Why More Women Should Enter Chiropractic

Chiropractic offers an outstanding career for a woman. Although at present one out of six chiropractors is a woman, the ratio of women to men students now enrolled in chiropractic colleges is one out of four. These percentages are higher than are found in the other health-care professions. Further, the percentage of women enrolled in chiropractic colleges is on the increase, whereas the percentage of women enrolled in medical colleges has not changed in the past half century.

Women Doctors of Chiropractic earn the same as male practitioners. Further, they receive the same prestige and opportunities. There seems to be less prejudice toward a woman Doctor of Chiropractic than toward female practitioners in many other health fields.

A woman does not have to possess great physical strength to be a chiropractor. Rather, patience and skill are more important.

Women have been successful in all areas of chiropractic from pediatrics to general practice. Some specialize in the health care of women.

Women are also active in areas other than private practice, such as research or teaching. Further opportunities abound in special clinics and industry.

Why Chiropractic Appeals to Women

Many women feel unfulfilled in performing the jobs they have chosen to escape from the boredom of household activities. In helping others to achieve better health, women find purpose; chiropractic is a prestigious profession that women find absorbing and challenging.

Few professions offer the freedom that chiropractic does. Thus it perfectly suits a married woman raising a family. She can practice her profession during hours that best suit her needs. For example, she may decide to open her office only three days a week or to see patients in the mornings only. The choice is hers alone. She can see as many or as few patients as she desires.

In some cases women practitioners have married fellow students or colleagues and set up a husband-wife office, a situation which is often ideal. Some women have done extremely well in the profession.

One of the best-known and most successful women chiropractors was the late Dr. Ruth R. Cleveland of Kansas City, Missouri, who was a cofounder of the Cleveland Chiropractic College. She was the student of another famous female chiropractor, Sylvia Ashworth of Nebraska.

Dr. Cleveland was licensed in four states, held numerous offices in chiropractic organizations, and was the editor of the official *Journal of the Missouri State Chiropractic Association*.

At Cleveland Chiropractic College she taught anatomy and dissection, and she was the director of the clinic there for nearly twenty years. After retiring from the college she became noted for her work in pediatrics.

Other notable women chiropractors include Dr. Dee Tweed, who holds three doctorates—a D.C., a D.M. and a Ph.D. She is chairperson of the Basic Science Department at Texas Chiropractic College. Dr. Carol Port, another successful woman chiropractor, practiced in Australia and South Africa before going to

Los Angeles Chiropractic College. Her patients have included members of the New South Wales rugby and polo teams and members of the Australian Ballet.

Another well-known practitioner, Dr. Mary Ann Pruitt, has practiced chiropractic with her father, Dr. Sterling Pruitt, for thirty-three years in Forth Worth, Texas. She has received numerous honors for outstanding service to the profession. She is a distinguished fellow of the ICA, was awarded the Ph.C. from Palmer College, and has been vice-president and secretary of the Chiropractic Society of Texas. She is now serving her second term as president of that organization. Married to Lewis Armstrong and the mother of two children, she is listed in *Who's Who in Texas.*

These are only a few of the many women who have made highly successful careers as chiropractors. Evidence of their success is everywhere. Presently, women are presidents of two of the ten national councils on chiropractic diagnosis and internal disorders: the Council on Mental Health and the Council of Women Chiropractors.

Comments from Successful Women Practitioners in Chiropractic

Probably the best insight a future chiropractor can get into what women actually feel about their profession is to ask them. Four women chiropractors told us of their feelings in this manner.

Dr. S. of New Jersey, who enjoys a successful practice says, "Chiropractic gives me a fulfillment and purpose in life which is second to none. I feel privileged to be among its practitioners."

Dr. P. of California, who has two assistants and three nurses working in her clinic, states, "The chiropractic profession has afforded me a life-style that would not have been available to me in another profession. Not only is there financial stability, but there is a sense of great achievement."

"I truly am grateful to my profession. It allows me to alleviate some of the pain and suffering in mankind," says Dr. A. of Florida, who maintains a large practice.

Dr. L. of Ohio, who has three offices within a 50-mile radius, states, "The practice of chiropractic is the greatest challenge in the world. It returns health to a person without the use of drugs. Everytime I get a person well, the gratification I feel is over-whelming."

CHAPTER XIV

Relationships With the Other Healing Arts

Because of more stringent chiropractic educational requirements and increased research that has proven the success of
chiropractic care, the relationship with the other healing-arts
professions has gradually become more cordial and somewhat
less competitive.

The American Medical Association has always been conserva-
tive. Thus, it has resisted the efforts of chiropractic and to a lesser
degree osteopathy to present other points of view. There has
been a constant battle between these schools of healing, creating
competition where there should be cooperation.

The reasons for this competition are complex. Perhaps a great
deal of it has to do with the fact that medicine is in the majority
and is somewhat older than the other two schools. Thus, there
is a tendency to accept the established healing art of medicine as
being correct and all others as being unorthodox or wrong.

Also, a tremendous amount of money is available to the AMA
both from its members (for medical doctors pay a substantial
fee to belong to the organization) and from the federal government. This money permits the waging of a strong propaganda
campaign whenever necessary.

The AMA has fought quacks and cultists to protect the public, which is admirable. Unfortunately, this sometimes puts the AMA in the position of ignoring every approach but the one that is politically sound for the majority of its members.

The ACA has gone on record against the "monopolistic attitude of the American Medical Association," which it asserts is "not in the best interests of the public's health and welfare."

Certainly in our democratic society we have always been proud of our diversity of opinion. That is why chiropractors are so greatly concerned that the public should be able to choose between alternatives in health care.

Generally the competitive feeling is one-sided, for few chiropractors spend time attacking the medical profession. Rather their interest lies in improving the standards and techniques of chiropractic.

Television and the motion-picture industry have turned the medical doctor into a glamorous creature. The drama of a physician's life obviously couldn't be what we see on the screen—yet people have come to accept the stereotype of an almost superhuman creature. In fact, we are surprised to find that in many other countries doctors have little of the prestige that we bestow upon them. In Eastern European countries, for example, the medical doctor has relatively low status.

The allopathic professional has been painted as most glamorous—particularly surgeons, for the use of technology and life-and-death decisions can be more dramatic in surgery. Chiropractic (and to some extent osteopathic) physicians are more concerned with maintaining natural balance, which takes time and patience and thus makes for less drama. Further, many of the ailments that chiropractors deal with are not dramatic in the sense that they are contagious like typhoid fever or unusual diseases such as Hansen's disease, and thus do not lend themselves to dramatic representation. If they did, and the chiropractic physicians became the subjects of film and television melodramas, then overnight much of the prejudice against chiropractic would be wiped out! But this would be sheer propaganda, and thoughtful practitioners wish to develop a sounder program of educating the public.

It has been only within the past five years that paraprofessionals have appeared in the oldest established healing-arts profession —medicine. As time develops, no doubt technicians and aides will be utilized in the field of chiropractic as well. Since the field is still young, it is difficult to predict what will eventually unfold.

It is quite possible that in the future the lines between the medical doctors and the chiropractic doctors will become less distinct and that there will be a greater interchange of services.

Perhaps because conventional hospital care has become so expensive, medical physicians have been reluctant to suggest that patients spend long periods of time waiting for the body to adjust and cure itself on its own. (Patients often stay twelve weeks or more at Spears Hospital.) Thus, there may be more incentive to use surgery rather than prescribe alternative methods because of this often overlooked fact. Most people who seek chiropractic care fear and wish to avoid surgery or wish to try alternative measures first.

With chiropractors and physicians working in conjunction, each will have to permit the other to use techniques in which he alone is expert. Just as dentists do not treat colonic disorders and internists do not set broken bones, so chiropractic, say some of its practitioners, will move toward becoming a specialty of the healing arts. Instead of being a general practitioner the chiropractor of the future may work only in highly specialized areas.

Referrals to the Other Professions

Just as the medical general practitioner seldom attempts to treat every case that comes before him, so the chiropractic physician also refers some of his cases to other health-care professionals. Within his own area he might refer a patient to a chiropractic specialist in roentgenology, who would take very specialized X-ray photographs.

Presently chiropractors also refer some of their patients to medical doctors (according to the ACA, about 85 percent do so). In turn, some medical doctors refer patients to chiropractors. The number will probably increase as time goes by, because of such studies as the one done by researchers at the University of Utah, who found the quality and effectiveness of chiropractic and medical health care to be equal in treating football back injuries and that patients preferred certain types of treatment by chiropractors in certain types of injuries.

Further studies in four states have indicated that chiropractic rather than medical treatment of industrial injuries has reduced costs of treatment, cost of compensation, and loss of work time. Further, workmen's disability and suffering were lessened.

Educating Other Healing-Arts Professionals

A major concern of chiropractic physicians is to educate practitioners of the other healing arts. Thus, chiropractors have been meeting with medical groups around the world attempting to explain their approach to health care. For example, in 1974 chiropractors took part in an international meeting of the National Institutes of Health, a renowned research organization. In 1973 Medicare and Medicaid permitted payment to chiropractors for health-care services. And in 1974 the U.S. Office of Education recognized the Council on Chiropractic Education as an accrediting agency for chiropractic colleges, making their degrees valid and permitting the colleges to be eligible for federal financial assistance.

Thus, you will note that most of the gains made by chiropractors have been in the past few years! Change is very difficult and takes a long time. In many ways the strides made by chiropractic in such a short period of time are nothing less than phenomenal.

As in every field, there are extremists of one sort or another who usually grab the headlines. So, too, the medical profession has had its share of sensational cases as well as any of the other healing arts. These cases should be taken for what they actually are—exceptions. If practicing chiropractors continue to stress research as they are now doing, if education requirements are continually upgraded as they now are being, and if the other healing arts are willing to approach the art of chiropractic with an open mind as they are now beginning to do, the future of chiropractic will be boundless.

CHAPTER XV

The Future in Chiropractic

Shortage of Chiropractors

Most knowledgeable authorities agree that the supply of chiropractic physicians is currently insufficient. Many also contend that even with increased chiropractic school productivity, the supply of doctors will continue to be insufficient to provide adequate health services to an expanding population—a population ever more demanding of a higher quality and intensity of health care.

This insufficiency of personnel is felt most strongly in rural and inner urban areas. The poor and the medically indigent have higher rates of disability and death than the rest of the population, a fact that can at least in part be attributed to the lack of qualified medical personnel.

Administrative aspects of health insurance, Medicare, Medicaid, and liability problems have invaded the physician's time. Medical technology and research present new treatment modalities that must be learned and applied. Under these increasing pressures, physicians have engaged in group practice and have hired auxiliary personnel to perform routine tasks in data collection.

The need for more chiropractors is acute. Public schools, guidance counselors, and the people who have been helped by chiropractic are urging the youth of this nation to enter the profession.

In addition, the job market for chiropractic paraprofessionals is promising. Chiropractic assistants are now being trained at some colleges. These parachiropractic professionals are educated in anatomy, physiology, and the basic sciences as well as in X-ray and in the use of instruments used in chiropractic. The student also works alongside the chiropractor in clinics. The chiropractic assistant degree (C.A.) is seen as a nine-month course. The ACA and the ICA are both examining the courses that have been developed in various sections of the country.

New Approaches

Chiropractic seems destined to develop new approaches. Although apparently little or no work has been done in the area, the growing problems of drug addiction should be a natural field for chiropractic care.

The modern chiropractor suggests that drugs are dangerous substances that should be handled with far more discretion than they are today—although he does not insist that they be totally banned. But through counseling and other techniques he might be able to dissuade addicts from drug use without resorting to methadone or similar substitutes.

Since the chiropractor is opposed to drugs, he might be able to achieve extraordinary success in this field.

In addition, some success has been had in treating mentally ill patients. This is an area in which chiropractors may wish to do research. Other new approaches are being developed in hospitals and clinics.

Chiropractic hospital care is presently limited. The Spears Hospital is the best known. Many patients who have had health problems that have persisted in spite of care through other healing-arts practitioners have gone to Spears Hospital as a last resort. In addition to chiropractic adjustment, patients at the hospital are given controlled nutritional diet, hydrotherapy, physiotherapy, massage, and accupressure. Although a newspaper published by the hospital carries constant testimonials by former patients, the hospital does not claim cures. It does indicate, however, that "gratifying results" have been obtained on a wide range of conditions such as bronchial ailments, multiple sclerosis, and rheumatism.

Although few chiropractors would attempt to claim such a wide range of results for their own practices, the hospital, like other healing-arts facilities, offers many methods not available in most offices. Further, the hospital offers specialists in particular areas.

Colleges also offer patient services through their clinics, which are used for instruction of students in chiropractic under the careful supervision of a licensed practitioner.

Since the earliest days, chiropractors have sought to help those who felt they were at the end of their rope—that there was no hope to alleviate their pain and misery, as is the case of most of the patients who seek the help of chiropractors today.

Since chiropractors have responded with tact and understanding and have tried to help their patients in an intelligent manner, their patients have in turn responded with great appreciation.

Chiropractic is attempting to clarify some basic scientific premises in addition to developing new approaches.

At the University of Colorado, a federal grant of $230,000 has been given to continue a project originally funded by the chiropractic profession. The study, "Scientific Research on the Fundamentals of Chiropractic," makes use of equipment like the million-volt electron microscope to study the visual properties of cells. Researchers also use aerospace and engineering techniques to study stress in the human spine.

Research studies of this nature help chiropractic to define itself more clearly. Much criticism of chiropractic is based on ideas developed eighty years ago and to which most modern chiropractors no longer adhere. Certainly no one would fault medical doctors for outdated practices that have been abandoned, nor should chiropractic be thus faulted. On the other hand, some of the basic premises have proved sound and have been built upon.

Professor C. H. Suh of the University of Colorado, head of the chiropractic research project, recently said, "We would like to see the improvement of the chiropractic technique itself . . . If we know why chiropractic is working, then we know how to improve . . . because it has tremendous potential in the future health care system."

Future Trends

The chairman of the CCE Commission on Accreditation, Orval L. Hidde, D.C., J.D., has suggested that in the future chiropractors may be on the staffs of hospitals and other public institutions, included in all public health care and insurance programs, involved in public health policy-making decisions, and recipients of research funds. Further, he foresees future chairs of chiropractic established in universities and a tenfold increase in demand for chiropractic services.

In accordance with the push toward improving education standards, the Foundation for Chiropractic Education and Research has made a total of more than $4,000,000 in grants to colleges. The grants made during the first year ran to $38,400 grants-in-aid to colleges only and now run to $350,000 and higher. This foundation was begun in 1945 as the Chiropractic Research Foundation, changed its name to Foundation for Accredited Education in 1958, and became the foundation for Chiropractic Education and Research in 1967.

The foundation is nonprofit. It is organized to receive gifts to support and upgrade chiropractic education, to assist colleges in their developmental programs to provide adequate facilities and equipment for the full and complete education of students, to provide chiropractic clinics, and to promote the science of chiropractic. It is organized exclusively for charitable scientific and educational purposes, with no part of the income or net earnings to be used for the benefit of any individual or to carry on propaganda or influence legislation.

Few blacks, Hispanics, and other ethnic minority-group members have entered chiropractic, although they are welcome to do so. Probably there has been little effort by counselors in high schools to interest students in this area, although many students are encouraged to go into the allied health fields. Also there may be a lack of financial resources to permit an interested student to enter the field. Further, public-school conditions often have been so poor that students are not sufficiently prepared in the sciences to permit them to achieve success.

Fortunately, the development of community colleges throughout the country with strong remedial programs may offer members of minority groups compensatory education to help them bridge the gap. Better counseling on all levels may point out the desirability of a chiropractic career to members of minority groups who might be interested in such a career.

Chiropractic Colleges

The following colleges have status with the Council on Chiropractic Education (the national accrediting association):

New York Chiropractic College   Accredited
P.O. Box 167
Glen Head, New York 11545

Logan College of Chiropractic   Accredited
1851 Schoettler Road
Chesterfield, St. Louis, Missouri 63017

Los Angeles College of Chiropractic   Accredited
16200 East Amber Valley Drive
Whittier, California 90609

National College of Chiropractic   Accredited
200 East Roosevelt Road
Lombard, Illinois 60148

Northwestern College of Chiropractic   Accredited
1834 Mississippi River Boulevard
St. Paul, Minnesota 55116

Palmer College of Chiropractic   Accredited
1095 Dunford Way
Sunnyvale, California 94087

Texas Chiropractic College   Accredited
5912 Spencer Highway
Pasadena, Texas 77505

Western States Chiropractic College   Accredited
2900 N.E. 132nd Avenue
Portland, Oregon 97230

Cleveland Chiropractic College   Accredited
6401 Rockhill Road
Kansas City, Missouri 64131

Recognized Candidates for Accreditation

Cleveland Chiropractic College
590 North Vermont Avenue
Los Angeles, California 90004

Life Chiropractic College
1269 Barclay Circle
Marietta, Georgia 30062

Pasadena College of Chiropractic
1505 North Marengo Avenue
Pasadena, California 91103

International College of Chiropractic
P.O. Box 96
Bundoora, Victoria 3083, Australia

The following affiliate members are foreign chiropractic colleges that subscribe to the policies and regulations of the Council:

Anglo-European College of Chiropractic
Cavendish Road
Bournemouth, England

Canadian Memorial Chiropractic College
1900 Bayview Avenue
Toronto, Ontario, Canada M4G3E6

APPENDIX B

National Organizations

The following are national associations to which many chiropractors belong. These two professional organizations offer students in chiropractic colleges the opportunity to become members.

American Chiropractic Association
2200 Grand Avenue
Des Moines, Iowa 50312

International Chiropractors Association
741 Brady Street
Davenport, Iowa 52808

A Typical Course of Instruction

Course No.	Course	Hours	Credits
	First Trimester		
10.30	Anatomy (Embryology)	64	2
10.81	Anatomy (Splanchnology)	48	1.5
10.41	Anatomy (Histology I)	80	2
10.70	Anatomy (Osteology & Orthopedy)	96	3
20.01	Physiology I	80	2.5
91.11	Palpation I	32	0.5
93.00	Chiropractic Philosophy	32	0.5
92.11	Principles, Basic I	32	1
91.20	Technic	16	0
		480	13.0
	Second Trimester		
10.10	Anatomy (Angiology)	48	1.5
10.51	Anatomy (Myology and Syndesmology I)	48	1.5
10.82	Anatomy (Splanchnology)	48	1.5
10.42	Anatomy (Histology II) (including Lab)	80	2
10.61	Anatomy (Neurology I)	32	1
20.02	Physiology I	64	2

Course No.	Course	Hours	Credits
91.12	Palpation II	32	0.5
92.21	Principles I	32	1
92.12	Principles, Basic II	32	1
91.31	Technic I	32	0.5
94.13	X-ray Marking	32	0.5
		480	13.0

Third Trimester

10.52	Anatomy (Myology & Syndesmology II)	64	2
10.62	Anatomy (Neurology II)	96	3
30.10	Inorganic Chemistry	80	2.5
60.01	Microbiology	48	1.5
50.01	Pathology	32	1
91.13	Palpation III	32	0.5
92.22	Principles II	32	1
92.41	Instrumentation I	32	0.5
91.32	Technic II	32	0.5
94.14	X-ray Interpretation	32	0.5
		480	13.0

Fourth Trimester

10.63	Anatomy (Neurology III)	96	3
30.21	Organic Chemistry I	32	1
70.11	Physical Diagnosis I	32	1
60.02	Microbiology II	32	1
50.02	Pathology II	32	1
20.03	Physiology III	64	2
91.41	Technic-Basic I	32	0.5
91.33	Technic III	32	0.5
92.42	Instrumentation II	32	0.5
94.15	Cervical X-ray Marking	32	0.5
01.11	Clinical Instruction I	32	1
94.11	X-ray Physics	32	1
		480	13.0

Course No.	Course	Hours	Credits
	Fifth Trimester		
10.64	Anatomy (Neurology IV)	32	1
10.20	Anatomy (Applied)	48	1.5
30.22	Organic Chemistry II	48	1.5
70.21	Laboratory Diagnosis I	32	1
70.12	Physical Diagnosis II	32	1
60.03	Microbiology III	64	2
50.03	Pathology III	32	1
20.04	Physiology IV	64	2
91.42	Technic-Basic II	32	0.5
94.16	Cervical X-ray Technic	32	0.5
01.12	Clinical Instruction II	32	1
94.12	X-ray Placement	32	1
		480	14.0
	Sixth Trimester		
30.31	Biochemistry I	64	2
70.22	Laboratory Diagnosis II	32	1
70.13	Physical Diagnosis III	48	1.5
60.04	Microbiology IV	64	2
50.04	Pathology IV	64	2
20.05	Physiology V	48	1.5
92.50	Spinal Abnormalities	32	1
80.05	Pediatrics	32	1
91.43	Technic-Basic III	32	0.5
91.51	Physiotherapy I	64	1
		480	13.5
	Seventh Trimester		
30.32	Biochemistry II	48	1.5
70.23	Laboratory Diagnosis III	64	2.0
70.14	Physical Diagnosis IV	48	1.5
80.21	Obstetrics	80	2.5
50.05	Pathology V	48	1.5
40.01	Public Health I	64	2

Course No.	Course	Hours	Credits
94.17	X-ray Pathology I	32	1
92.31	Chiropractic Science I	32	1
91.52	Physiotherapy II	64	1
		480	14.0

Eighth Trimester

30.33	Biochemistry III	48	1.5
70.24	Laboratory Diagnosis IV	48	1.5
70.15	Physical Diagnosis V	48	1.5
80.01	Dietetics	32	1
80.22	Gynecology	80	2.5
50.06	Pathology VI	64	2
80.11	Psychology I	32	1
40.02	Public Health II	32	1
94.18	X-ray Pathology II	48	1.5
92.32	Chiropractic Science II	32	1
91.63	Technic-Auxiliary III	16	0.5
		480	15.0

Ninth Trimester

70.25	Laboratory Diagnosis V	32	1
80.02	Dermatology	32	1
70.16	Physical Diagnosis VI (Endocrinology)	64	2
80.03	Geriatrics	32	1
50.07	Pathology VII	32	1
80.12	Psychology II	32	1
40.03	Public Health III	48	1.5
80.04	Toxicology	32	1
92.33	Chiropractic Science III	32	1
92.60	First Aid	32	0.5
92.70	Office Procedure/Jurisprudence	32	0.5
92.43	Instrumentation III	48	0.5
91.64	Technic-Auxiliary IV	48	0.5
		480	12.5

Course No.	Course	Hours	Credits
	Required Externship		
01.31	Externship I	60	—
	(Taken during the 6th Trimester)		
01.21	Externship II	240	3
	(Taken during the 7th Trimester)		
01.22	Externship III	240	3
	(Taken during the 8th Trimester)		
01.23	Externship IV	240	3
	(Taken during the 9th Trimester)		
01.32	Externship V	60	—
	(Taken after the 9th Trimester)		
		840	9.0
	Total Number of Hours and Credits	5,160	130.5

APPENDIX D

Educational Requirements for Licensure

As of Feb. 1, 1977

UNITED STATES

Jurisdiction	Nonprofessional Education Required	Professional Education Required	Type of Examining Board
Alabama	High School	4 yrs. of 9 mo. each	†C
Alaska	H. S. & 2 yrs. College	4 yrs. of 9 mo. each	†C
Arizona	H. S. & 2 yrs. College	4 yrs. of 9 mo. each—4,000 hours	†C
Arkansas	H. S. & 2 yrs. College (1)	4 yrs. of 9 mo. each—4,400 hours	†C-B
California	H. S. & 2 yrs. College	4 yrs. of 9 mo. each	C
Colorado	High School	4 yrs.—4,000 hours	†C-B
Connecticut	H. S. & 2 yrs. College	4 yrs. of 8 mo. each—4,000 hours	†C
Delaware	H. S. & 2 yrs. College	4 yrs. of 9 mo. each	†C
Dist. of Columbia	H. S. & 2 yrs. College	4 yrs. of 9 mo. each	†C-B
Florida	H. S. & 2 yrs. College	4 yrs.—4,200 hours	†C
Georgia	H. S. & 2 yrs. College	4 yrs. of 9 mo. each	†C
Hawaii	H. S. & 2 yrs. College	4 yrs. of 9 mo. each—4,200 hours	†C
Idaho	H. S. & 2 yrs. College	4 yrs. of 8 mo. each	†C
Illinois	H. S. & 2 yrs. College	4 yrs. of 8 mo. each	MX
Indiana	H. S. & 2 yrs. College	4 yrs.—4,000 hours	MX
Iowa	H. S. & 2 yrs. College	4 yrs.—4,000 hours	†C
Kansas	H. S. & 2 yrs. College	4 yrs. of 9 mo. each	†MX
Kentucky	H. S. & 2 yrs. College	4 yrs. of 9 mo. each—4,000 hours	†C
Louisiana	H. S. & 2 yrs. College	4 yrs.—4,000 hours	†C
Maine	H. S. & 2 yrs. College (2)	4 yrs.—4,400 hours	†C
Maryland	H. S. & 2 yrs. College	4 yrs.—4,000 hours	C
Massachusetts	H. S. & 2 yrs. College (3)	4 yrs.—4,000 hours	†MX
Michigan	H. S. & 2 yrs. College	4 yrs. of 9 mo. each—4,000 hours	†C

Educational Requirements for Licensure (continued)
UNITED STATES

Jurisdiction	Nonprofessional Education Required	Professional Education Required	Type of Examining Board
Minnesota	H. S. & 2 yrs. College	4 yrs. of 8 mo. each	†C
Mississippi	H. S. & 2 yrs. College	4 yrs. of 9 mo. each	†C
Missouri	High School	4 yrs. of 9 mo. each—4,000 hours	†C
Montana	H. S. & 2 yrs. College	4 yrs. of 9 mo. each—4,000 hours	†C
Nebraska	High School	4 yrs.—4,000 hours	†C
Nevada	H. S. & 2 yrs. College	4 yrs.—4,000 hours	†C
New Hampshire	High School	4 yrs. of 9 mo. each	†MX
New Jersey	H. S. & 2 yrs. College	4 yrs. of 4,000 hours	†C
New Mexico	H. S. & 2 yrs. College (4)	4 yrs. of 8 mo. each—4,000 hours	MX
New York	H. S. & 2 yrs. College (5)	4 yrs. of 9 mo. each	†C
North Carolina	H. S. & 2 yrs. College	4 yrs. of 8 mo. each—4,000 hours	†C
North Dakota	H. S. & 2 yrs. College (1)	4 yrs. of 9 mo. each—4,000 hours	†C
Ohio	H. S. & 2 yrs. College	4 yrs. of 9 mo. each—4,150 hours	†C
Oklahoma	H. S. & 2 yrs. College	4 yrs. of 9 mo. each—4,000 hours	†C
Oregon	H. S. & 2 yrs. College	4 yrs. of 9 mo. each—4,000 hours	†C
Pennsylvania	H. S. & 1 yr. College (6)	4 yrs. of 9 mo. each—4,000 hours	†C
Puerto Rico	H. S. & 2 yrs. College	4 yrs. of 9 mo. each	†C
Rhode Island	H. S. & 2 yrs. College	4 yrs. of 9 mo. each	C
South Carolina	H. S. & 2 yrs. College	4 yrs. of 9 mo. each	†C
South Dakota	H. S. & 2 yrs. College	4 yrs. of 9 mo. each	†C
Tennessee	H. S. & 2 yrs. College	4 yrs. of 8 mo. each	†C-B
Texas	H. S. & 1 yr. College	4 yrs. of 8½ mo. ea.—4,000 hours	†C-B†
Utah	H. S. & 2 yrs. College	4 yrs.—4,400 hours	†C
Vermont	H. S. & 2 yrs. College	4 yrs. of 8 mo. each	MX†
Virginia	H. S. & 2 yrs. College (7)	4,000 hours	†C-B†
Washington	H. S. & 2 yrs. College	4 yrs. of 9 mo. each—4,000 hours	†C
West Virginia	H. S. & 2 yrs. College	4 yrs. of 9 mo. each	†C
Wisconsin	H. S. & 2 yrs. College	4 yrs. of 9 mo. each	†C
Wyoming	H. S. & 2 yrs. College	4 yrs. of 9 mo. each	†C

CANADA

Alberta	Junior Matriculation (8)	4 yrs. of 8 mo. each	*C
British Columbia	1 yr. Canadian College or equivalent	4 yrs. of 8 mo. each	*C
Manitoba	Junior Matriculation	4 academic years	
New Brunswick	Senior Matriculation	4 yrs. of 9 mo. each	*C
Ontario	Grade XIII	4 yrs. of 9 mo. each—4,200 hours	*C
Prince Edward Island	Grade XIII	Approved college	
Saskatchewan	Senior Matriculation	4 yrs. of 8 mo. each	*C
Nova Scotia	No information		*C
Quebec	No information		*C

Symbols designating Boards: C—Chiropractic. C-B—Chiropractic & Basic Science. MX—Mixed (Compound of medical and chiropractic members).

† Recognize or utilize National Board of Chiropractic Examiners Certificate. (Some additional states consider on an individual basis)
* Recognize examinations of Canadian Chiropractic Examining Board.

(1) Must include the basic sciences.
(2) Must include English and biology.
(3) Should include six semester hours of biology, chemistry, or physics.
(4) After January 1, 1976, except for those previously enrolled.
(5) Must include six semester hours each in English, physics, biology or zoology, general chemistry, and three semester hours of organic chemistry.
(6) Must include six semester hours each in chemistry, biology, and physics.
(7) For those matriculating on or after January 1, 1975.
(8) A Junior Matriculation Certificate or its equivalent is equal to a high-school diploma or its equivalent.

Reprinted courtesy of the Department of Education of the American Chiropractic Association, 2200 Grand Avenue, Des Moines, Iowa 50312

APPENDIX E

Educational Requirements
of Non-American Chiropractic Associations

Foreign applicants from countries represented by the Associations in the following list must present a letter of approval from the corresponding organization to be considered for enrollment.

Country	Requirements	Contact
Australia	1. In order to obtain a scholarship an applicant must possess a certificate that will entitle him to enter any Australian university. 2. In order to obtain endorsement students must have successfully completed five years of secondary education. If an applicant receives endorsement of a state branch and has not sufficient secondary education, he must agree to upgrade his education to the required standard prior to or concurrent with his chiropractic education by attending an approved junior college.	H. C. Rutledge, D.C. Secretary Queensland Branch, ACA 2687 Gold Coast Highway Broadbeech, Queensland 4217 S. J. Bardsley, D.C. Secretary Victoria Branch, ACA 36 Main Street Mornington, Victoria 3931 N. O. Martin, D.C. Secretary N.S.W. Branch, ACA 136 Willoughby Road Crow's Nest New South Wales 5231

A. E. Minty, D.C.
Secretary
W. A. Branch, ACA
872 Albany Highway
East Victoria Park
Western Australia 6101

J. E. Longbottom, D.C.
Secretary
S. A. Branch, ACA
75 Gawler Street
Mt. Barker
South Australia 5231

Belgium

1. A curriculum vitae.
2. A certificate of good standing and behavior.
3. Diploma of "Humanities completes," dument homologue certificate of two years of "Candidature en sciences naturelle et medicale."
4. The chiropractic studies to be completed in four years of nine months each in four separate calendar years.

Dr. John Gillet
Vice-president
Association des Chiropracticiens
Belges
5, rue de La Limite
Bruxelles 3, Belgium

Denmark

1. Certificate of the "Studentes Eksamen" (Danish).
2. Certificate confirming this on a formular signed by the Chairman of the Danish Chiropractors' Council.

Dr. Svend Nielsen
Chairman
Danish Chiropractors' Association
Sdr. Boulevard 14
Maribo, Denmark

Educational Requirements of Non-American Chiropractic Associations (continued)

Country	Requirements	Contact
England	1. At least four passes in the General Certificate of Education at "ordinary" (o) level. 2. One pass in a science subject at "advanced" (a) level—preferably zoology (alternate: physics or chemistry). 3. Pass at "o" level or its near two science subjects named above. 4. The British Association requests the opportunity to interview the prospective students before their acceptance by the college.	Winston Brownrigg, D.C. Hon. Secretary Mountpottinger House The Mount Belfast 5, England Tel. Belfast 57919
France	1. Certificate of the first "Baccalaureat" 2. Certificate of the second "Baccalaureat"	Dr. Henri Schmoukler 79 rue D'Amsterdam Paris 8, France
Italy	1. Qualifications for university entrance	Dr. F. Grillo, Secretary European Chiropractors Union Zuchwilerstasse 10 4500 Solothurn Switzerland Tel. 065 2 91 21
Japan		Kazuyoshi Takeyachi, D.C. President Japanese Chiropractic Society 9-5-3 Chrome Kitaaoyama Minato-Ku Tokyo, Japan

Norway	1. Certificate of Matriculation 2. "Examen Philosophicum"	Halvor Sorbye, D.C. Norwegian Chiropractic Association Gamle Drammensvei 48 1320 Stabekk, Norway
South Africa & Rhodesia	University entrance certificate or equivalent	L. Fisher Honorable National Secretary Chiropractic Association of South Africa 902, Metro Centre Bree Street Johannesburg, South Africa Tel. 22–7772
Sweden	1. Certificate of Student-examen, also called Mogensetsexamen. This is the equivalent of high school and two years of junior college in the United States.	Arvid Andren, D.C. President The Swedish Chiropractic Society Olandsgatan 8 38100 Kalmar Sweden
Switzerland	1. Certificate of the "Matura" 2. The commercial "maturiat" diploma is not valid since January 1965. Only diploma types A, B, and C. 3. According to the new law for the protection against ionizing radiation, the chiropractors have to pass a federal examination on nuclear physics, physics of roentgenology, human genetics, radiation hazards, and protection against roentgen radiation.	Dr. Bruno J. Widmann President Swiss Chiropractic Association Rathausgasse 9, Aarau Switzerland

Educational Requirements of Non-American Chiropractic Associations (continued)

Country	Requirements	Contact
Other European Countries		Dr. F. Grillo, Secretary European Chiropractors Union Zuchwilerstrasse 10 4500 Solothurn Switzerland Tel. 065 2 91 21

Courtesy: International Chiropractors Association, 741 Brady Street, Davenport, Iowa 52808

ACA Policies on Public Health and Related Matters

ACUPUNCTURE

The Board of Governors of the ACA encourages the judicious development of curriculae, research, and clinical procedures of this ancient healing method, and that it be integrated, when appropriate, as an adjunctive and supportive procedure which may complement the chiropractic adjustment. This modality should be utilized only by the doctor of chiropractic who is qualified by education and clinical experience, and who has been examined and certified by an appropriate accredited body.

The Board suggests a minimal curricula as the following: (a) 200 hours of study under institutions having status with the Council on Chiropractic Education or appropriately recognized instructors; (b) 100 hours of clinical application, including at least 10 case reports, fully documented and researched; and (c) Examination by an institution and/or licensing board in clinical and didactic aspects. (Ratified by the House of Delegates June 1975.)

AMERICAN MEDICAL ASSOCIATION

Resolved, that the ACA is opposed to unnecessary compulsory medication, unnecessary surgery, and the arbitrary monopolistic attitude of the American Medical Association which is not in the best interests of the public's health and welfare. (Ratified by the House of Delegates June 1966.)

CERTIFICATION PROGRAMS

The ACA supports and abides by The Council on Chiropractic Education policy on specialty certification and recognizes that the specialty councils, not the colleges, are engaged in such programs. (Approved July 1975.)

CHIROPRACTIC DEFINITION

Chiropractic is that science and art which utilizes the inherent recuperative powers of the body and the relationship between the musculoskeletal structures and functions of the body, particularly of the spinal column and the nervous system, in the restoration and maintenance of health. (ACA Master Plan ratified by the House of Delegates June 1964, amended June 1975.)

CHIROPRACTIC DISCIPLINES

Resolved, that the American Chiropractic Association reject any attempt inside or outside the profession to lock our discipline into any static a priori positions, be they past, present or future. (Ratified by the House of Delegates July 1974.)

CHIROPRACTIC PRACTICES AND PROCEDURES

The practices and procedures which may be employed by doctors of chiropractic are based on the academic and clinical training received in and through accredited chiropractic colleges. These shall include, but are not limited to, the use of diagnostics and therapeutics, specifically including the adjustment and manipulation of the articulations and adjacent tissues of the human body, particularly of the spinal column; included is the treatment of intersegmental disorders for alleviation of related neurological aberrations. Patient care is conducted with due regard for environmental, nutritional, and psychotherapeutic factors, as well as first aid, hygiene, sanitation, rehabilitation and physiological therapeutic procedures designed to assist in the restoration and maintenance of neurological integrity and homeostatic balance. (ACA Master Plan, ratified by the House of Delegates June 1964, amended June 1975.)

CHIROPRACTIC PRINCIPLE

Chiropractic is based on the premise that the relationship between structure and function in the human body is a significant health factor and that such relationships between the spinal column and the nervous system are the most significant, since the normal transmission and expression of nerve energy are essential to the restoration and maintenance of health. (ACA Master Plan, ratified by the House of Delegates June 1964, amended June 1975.)

COMPREHENSIVE HEALTH-CARE BENEFITS

Another major national health goal should be the provision to all Americans of the whole spectrum of comprehensive health-care benefits, including ambulatory, preventive and rehabilitative services. The goal should be provision of the services of all licensed health-care providers, including dental, chiropractic, optometric, and mental health to name but a few of the health-care services which are often ignored in such health planning. The comprehensiveness of the services should encompass all the services authorized by all licensed health-care providers and not be limited to hospital-oriented services . . . The United States must have a system oriented to maintaining good health and avoiding illness, not merely one that waits until sickness has already occurred . . . Good health requires a system that provides comprehensive health care, preventive health care, and health maintenance.

Inclusion of chiropractic in such a comprehensive benefit

structure would be consistent with the precedent already enacted in Medicare and the Federal Employees Compensation Act as well as under the Internal Revenue Code where Federal income-tax deductions are authorized for expenditure for chiropractic care in the same manner as for "medical" care. The American Chiropractic Association urges that comprehensiveness of program benefits requires the availability of all licensed health services, including prevention and early detection, care and treatment, and rehabilitation. (Guidelines for National Health Planning Goals, approved November 1975.)

CONTINUING EDUCATION PROGRAMS

Resolved, that the ACA request the Council on Chiropractic Education join the American Chiropractic Association in a petition to the Federation of Chiropractic Licensing Boards seeking a uniform approval procedure for continuing education and convention programs conducted under the auspices of the CCE and its member institutions for the purpose of license renewal. (Ratified by the House of Delegates July 1974.)

The ACA supports the position of the Council on Chiropractic Education on continuing education which states in part, "The Council holds that only academic institutions can and should conduct postgraduate courses and deplores the itinerant, privately conducted programs generally presented for private gain."

The ACA subscribes to and recommends the Educational Standard for Postgraduate (Continuing) Education of The Council on Chiropractic Education. (Approved July 1975.)

COOPERATION WITH SCIENTIFIC COMMUNITY

Resolved, in the spirit of the NINDS Conference, the ACA stands ready to cooperate with the scientific community in the delivery of chiropractic as a valid health service to the benefit of the citizens of the United States and throughout the world. (Ratified by the House of Delegates June 1975.)

DANGERS OF UNQUALIFIED ADJUSTING

Resolved, that the ACA inform the American public that there are inherent dangers in the misuse of the manipulative adjustment by persons other than those adequately trained and qualified by due educational and examination process. (Ratified by the House of Delegates July 1971.)

DEPARTMENT OF EDUCATION

The ACA Board of Governors and the Foundation for Chiropractic Education and Research (FCER) trustees agree that the Department of Education will be a function of FCER effective April 1, 1971. FCER will assume responsibility for salaries, payroll taxes, and travel. ACA will provide office space and expense items outlined in the Department of Education section of the 1971–1972 budget. FCER will provide support funds for the Council on Chiropractic Education (CCE). (Approved January 1971.)

DIAGNOSIS

When a doctor of chiropractic clinically observes a condition in a patient, he seeks to find out "Why?", just as is done in physics, chemistry, and medicine. After such clinical observations are made, an attempt is made to explain the condition by a hypothesis. Such hypotheses are found in chiropractic literature under the heading of "Chiropractic Principles or Philosophy," but they are chiropractic hypotheses.

The probability or nonprobability of the hypothesis does not alter the chiropractic clinical facts, for the hypothesis is simply an interim attempt to explain the etiology of the clinical fact.

Chiropractic treats the ailment disclosed by the clinical facts, not by hypothesis. The patient's needs are met by the clinical efficacy of chiropractic, not by conflicting arguments on hypothesis.

Every chiropractic college teaches physical examination and diagnostic procedures and examines (or tests) in physical, clinical, laboratory, and differential analysis, in addition to chiropractic analysis. Before receiving a license to practice chiropractic, candidates are examined in diagnosis either by official state boards or by the National Board of Chiropractic Examiners, or both.

The chiropractic curriculum is oriented toward patient management, that is, to the recognition of the measures best suited to the restoration and maintenance of the patient's good health (whether such measures are applied by a doctor of chiropractic or by another health professional on referral).

Present-day chiropractic does not hold that the subluxation is the only cause of disease. Whatever may have been said in chiropractic literature years ago, today's chiropractic education and practice recognizes multiple causes of, and multiple methods of treatment for, disease.

The doctor of chiropractic must first evaluate the needs of the patient before administering any type of care. If he should determine that the case is within his scope, he proceeds to provide appropriate care. But if he determines that the patient requires another type of care, he refers the patient to that method which he believes is most advantageous. (Chiropractic White Paper, May 1969, Board approved July 1975.)

DISASSOCIATION WITH CULTISM

Resolved, that the ACA disassociate itself from cultism and trade practices in keeping with the standards and conduct of a scientific branch of the healing arts, and shall sever all bonds of association or activity which would detract from our identification with scientific objectives. (Ratified by the House of Delegates June 1965.)

DISASSOCIATION WITH MONO-CAUSAL CONCEPTS

Resolved, that the House of Delegates officially clarify its position and disaffirm the doctrine that holds to a singular approach to the treatment of disease. (Ratified by the House of Delegates June 1975.)

DISTRIBUTION OF NATIONAL HEALTH SERVICES

Federal support of health programs should be geared to a decentralization of health-care facilities through a program of regional health centers which should provide the full range of state-licensed health services, to be available at the patient's free choice. This system of regional health centers should be supplemented by a system of helicopter or surface ambulances with fast service to major hospitals, where necessary.

In order to augment the availability of often unused health-care provider services, there should be a more widespread use of a broadened range of health-care services, including clinically effective therapies such as psychiatry, dentistry, chiropractic, home nursing, etc., in (a) all Federally sponsored health programs, including HMOs, and (b) all existing Federally operated or Federally supported health programs (including such as VA, CHAMPUS, Armed Services health programs, Federal employee benefit program, Longshoremen's and Harbor Worker's Compensation program, etc.), and in all future Federally operated and sponsored programs.

The Federal Government should adopt a program of increasing ambulatory and outpatient care, where professionally desirable, in all Federal and Federally sponsored health programs, including the use of the full range of licensed health professions (such as chiropractic, for example). (Guidelines for National Health Planning Goals, approved November 1975.)

EARTH DAY

Resolved, that the ACA does pledge support to "Earth Day" and such other public health endeavors as may arise. (Ratified by the House of Delegates June 1970.)

FACTORS OF GOOD HEALTH

Good health is not the equivalent of medical or health care for sickness. The health-care system is not the only factor which affects or determines the nation's health . . . Good health depends on other factors such as (1) good housing and proper sanitary facilities, including waste water disposal and garbage removal; (2) good nutrition, including safe and healthful foods; (3) good public environment, including freedom from air and water pollution, from toxic chemicals, and from communicable diseases; (4) good working environment, including freedom from exposures to industrial accidents and occupational health hazards; (5) good life-style, including freedom from deleterious effects of smoking, drugs, and alcohol, and reduction of traffic accidents and injuries . . . (6) good health attitudes and widespread use of preventive health-care techniques and facilities.

In the long run, factors such as above outlined, and others, may be more important health programs than health-care delivery itself, and the nation's health-care delivery system must be developed for appropriate coordination with all these factors affecting good health. Thus, good health is broader than the health-care industry itself. Furthermore, good health is not dependent upon the control of any one segment of the health-care industry over the other participants. The health-care industry must not be subject to the monopoly of medical doctors; all licensed health-care providers (including Doctors of Chiropractic) must be regarded as having a valid role to play in that health-care delivery system, to the degree of their licensed authority. (Guidelines for National Health Planning Goals, approved November 1975.)

FEDERAL FUNDING OF RESEARCH, EDUCATION, AND OTHER RELATED PROGRAMS

Chiropractic should be included in Federal funding of research, education scholarships and fellowships, health manpower training, construction of teaching, library and other facilities, and other related grant programs available to other health-care professions under Federal law. Federal grants and other funds are available to medical schools, and other related health-care institutions, as well as to students and researchers in those fields. Almost NONE of this is now available to chiropractic. Thus, while the substantial portion of funding for other health areas is Federal in research, scholarships and fellowships; health manpower training construction programs; aid for faculty salaries, libraries and school maintenance in one form or another, among other major Federal forms of financing of health-care professions, chiropractic has had to pay its own way out of private funds.

Provision of Federal funds for chiropractic in the same manner as provided to other health-care professions, such as medicine, is solely a question of fairness to and health protection for the American people. It is in the public interest that users of chiropractic health care profit from the same help as is made available to users of other forms of health care. Improving chiropractic health care and the chiropractic delivery system is as important to those who use its services as improving medicine's delivery system is to users of its services. Both are legally authorized health-care services, and the American taxpayers who prefer chiropractic health care should not be denied the aid that can come from Federal funds while other taxpayers who use medicine or other forms of health care can profit from such aid.

This is discriminatory tax policy, is contrary to the best interests of the American people, and is deleterious to the advancement and improvement of the public health. Therefore, chiropractic should be included in the Federal funding of its programs to the same extent as other health-care groups are funded by Federal funds. (Guidelines for National Health Planning Goals, approved November 1975.)

FEES, CASE BASIS

Case basis fees are not usual and customary in the chiropractic profession and recommendations should be made accordingly. There is no known currently acceptable statistical basis for computation of a "case basis" fee for chiropractic services. It is advised that the chiropractic physician may assume unnecessary legal risks when participating in this type of contractual relationship, and there may be implied warranty, despite contractual language disclaiming such. It is the position of the ACA that third-party payors and/or patients are within their rights to require itemization of services rendered. (Approved July 1975.)

FEES, PROFESSIONAL SERVICE

The ACA holds the position that professional fees charged by the chiropractic physician and paid by the patient are a part of the doctor-patient relationship and does not advise nor condone interference with this relationship or other contractual relationships of the respective parties.

Reimbursement where third-party contracts call for reimbursement on the basis of usual, customary, and reasonable should be consistent with the customary fees of the profession in a given geographical and/or socioeconomic area.

Current reimbursement policy for chiropractic services under Medicare is not consistent with customary chiropractic practice. Such policy creates an economic hardship for the Medicare recipient and deprives the recipient of the greater benefits which are available through customary chiropractic diagnostic and therapeutic procedures. (Approved July 1975.)

FEES, UNIT BASIS

Unit basis fees are not usual and customary in the chiropractic profession and recommendations should be made accordingly. It is the position of the ACA that unit pricing calls for detailed justification for the medical necessity for each unit of care given. (Approved July 1975.)

FREEDOM OF CHOICE IN HEALTH CARE

The American system is characterized by a free competitive economy, in which the public is free to choose to the maximum extent possible in the circumstancs among providers of products and services who compete for the public's patronage . . . This freedom of choice by the American purchaser is the hallmark of the American free competitive system which has brought this country to greatness, affluence, and the highest standard of living ever known to organized society.

Chiropractic recommends that Congress guaranty the consumer his freedom of choice of health-care provider, both in principle and in fact, as an iron-bound right. Only in this way can any national health goal be truly responsive to the American health-consumer's needs and demands. The consumer's freedom of choice, to select among all State-licensed health-care providers, is an essential attribute of any effective and responsive national health goals. By whatever statutory means seem appropriate and necessary, the American health consumer should be guaranteed his right to obtain chiropractic services and all other licensed health services in any national health goals. (Guidelines for National Health Planning Goals, approved November 1975.)

HEALTH-CARE SERVICES ELIGIBILITY AND ACCESS

A paramount goal of any national health planning and development should be a universal eligibility for health care, through comprehensive coverage of all the people of the United States, regardless of income. Therefore, in the judgment of the American Chiropractic Association, the first priority of national health goals should be an assurance of access to proper and adequate health care for everyone in the nation, regardless of their wealth or poverty. Anything less would be a denial to Americans of their basic right to obtain necessary health care . . . The health-care crisis facing the average American, whether resident in the big cities or in the rural countryside, is inability to obtain health care when and where needed at an affordable cost.

The development of national health goals obviously involves a search for analysis of alternatives. Chiropractic represents a legally sanctioned alternative, at least in part, to allopathic and osteopathic health. Therefore, a meaningful inventory of health-care alternatives which is basic to a policy decision on national health goals must include a full exploration and funding of chiropractic if a potential and valuable alternative is not to be ignored.

Therefore, the American Chiropractic Association urges that the very first national health goal should be a statutory guaranty to every American of the right of access to all licensed health services (including chiropractic), irrespective of the level of his income. (Guidelines for National Health Planning Goals, approved November 1975.)

HEALTH FREEDOM

Resolved, that monopoly of drug-oriented doctors in the public health field be discontinued so that parity and equal treatment be accorded to all licensed healing arts. Fair representation be established on all public health boards, commissions, and committees for all licensed branches of the healing arts. All members of all licensed healing arts shall have equal access to the use of the facilities of all tax-supported health institutions. (Ratified by the House of Delegates June 1972.)

INCLUSION IN FEDERAL HEALTH-CARE PROGRAMS

Chiropractic health care should be available, on a free choice basis, in all forms and organizations of health care provided directly by the Federal Government or financed in whole or in part out of Federal funds.

The American people should have the right of Freedom of Choice, under Federal or Federally financed health-care programs, to the services of a doctor of chiropractic licensed by the state where the service is provided. The right of the American people to such State-licensed health-care services is now denied in a variety of Federal programs, such as (for example) (1) veterans medical programs, (2) military medical programs, (3) CHAMPUS, (4) civilian medical programs of the Public Health Service, (5) regional medical health centers, and (6) special Federal programs such as Longshoremen's Harbor Workers' Compensation Act.

In addition, although chiropractic is included in Medicare and Medicaid, the allowable services are but a portion of those authorized under chiropractic licensing laws. Medicare, Medicaid, and future national health insurance coverage of chiropractic health-care services should be co-terminous with that authorized by State licensing laws, and Federal law should be revised (or passed) to provide accordingly. (Guidelines for National Health Planning Goals, approved November 1975.)

Chiropractic should be included in the mainstream of the nation's health care system not only by being included in Federal health-care delivery systems, and research and other programs as recommended, but also by being treated as an equal partner among health-care professions. (Guidelines for National Health Planning Goals, approved November 1975.)

INFORMED CONSENT

Informed consent is generally applied, from a legal standpoint, when measuring the degree of responsibility and/or liability of a doctor in malpractice cases. In other words, the fact that a patient submits to treatment and does so voluntarily does not in itself lessen the liability of the doctor.

Today, the stand by which the doctor is judged is that of "informed consent." By that is meant, to what degree has the patient been informed of all of the potential consequences, dangers, and other factors, so that his consent is given with full knowledge of the inherent dangers to which he is exposed. Full knowledge in this sense could be construed as "informed consent" and would relieve the doctor of much liability as there would be an assumption of the risk on the part of the patient.

The concept of "informed consent" can also be applied to other contractual relationships such as those for examination and treatment which are everyday occurrences in the doctor's office. (Approved July 1975.)

INSURANCE CONTRACT EXCLUSIONS

The ACA is opposed to the contractual exclusions of diagnosis and manipulation of subluxation as presently written into various insurance contracts. The ACA Insurance Committee is directed to pursue every conciliatory and/or legal means to alleviate these restrictive contract riders without compromise of cost, peer review, or physician responsibility to his patient. (Approved February 1975.)

INTRAPROFESSIONAL POLICY

The American Chiropractic Association accepts all the responsibilities to society that are required of the chiropractic profession. ACA reaffirms its position that chiropractic must be preserved as a separate and distinct branch of the healing arts.

The position of the American Chiropractic Association is as originally established and annually reaffirmed that the individual Doctor of Chiropractic has the privilege and the obligation to practice in accordance with his education received in a recognized college of chiropractic and in accordance with the statutes of the state in which he practices.

The American Chiropractic Association extends an open invitation to meet with any other chiropractic group or organization to discuss, in accord with the statements above, those other items upon which they feel compelled to negotiate agreement in order to achieve a unified profession.

The American Chiropractic Association will continue its program for greater recognition and acceptance of the profession to the ultimate benefit of health service to the public and Doctors of Chiropractic everywhere.

The American Chiropractic Association will continue to work with and aid all state associations to develop their individual programs.

The American Chiropractic Association believes this is the best course for professional progress and invites all Doctors of Chiropractic to unite in this effort. (Adopted by the House of Delegates June 1967, reaffirmed June 1975.)

INTENSIVE DAY CARE

The ACA agrees with the Ad Hoc Intensive Day-Care Committee Report. Intensive Care (day care) is not a usual or customary procedure in the practice of chiropractic and recommendations should be made in accordance with recommendations from the Ad Hoc Intensive Day-Care Committee with addition of the following considerations: (a) Intensive Day Care is not a new procedure in health care; (b) Fees for services rendered within the facility are separate from facilities charges; and (c) All services rendered must be justifiable by the treating physician as medically necessary.

The ACA recognizes that in addition to usual chiropractic management, there are instances where there is justifiable medical necessity for retention of a patient for a limited period of time in order to more adequately perform diagnostic and/or therapeutic services. As with usual chiropractic procedures, substantiation for necessity of this type of management is the responsibility of the treating physician. (Approved July 1975.)

MEDICAL NECESSITY

Third-party contracts usually call for a direct relationship between covered services and medical necessity. There is also much concern in this area by federal and state legislators, particularly as it pertains to quality assurance and professional standards review organizations. The ACA agrees that there should be a responsible position relative to this by our profession and has researched the subject as it is understood by numerous of the third-party payors.

The ACA position refers to those appropriate examinations, therapeutic substances, and treatment procedures that are used by licensed practitioners to diagnose and treat patients with a specific condition. Implied is the fact that the condition be a recognized one and that the examinations, tests, therapeutic substances, and treatment procedures used are based on scientific principles ánd studies, are generally accepted by the profession as being needed, essential, and appropriate to properly diagnose and treat patients with the particular condition. Quality and quantity of examination and therapeutic procedures must be within the norms and/or criteria established by the profession as a whole for such a condition. Implied also is the fact that there must be documentation in the medical records and/or reports to substantiate the need for the services rendered. (Approved July 1975.)

MEDICARE

A joint statement of the American Chiropractic Association and the International Chiropractors Association submitted to the Subcommittee on Health, Committee on Ways and Means,

House of Representatives on Medicare, concluded that if the ACA/ICA recommendations are adopted, the following legislative changes would result: (1) the authorization of the payment to beneficiaries for X-rays performed or required by Doctors of Chiropractic and for physical examination (and related routine laboratory tests) for the purpose of determining subluxations and/or referral to other health care providers; (2) the authorization for Doctors of Chiropractic to demonstrate the existence of spinal subluxations by "other chiropractic procedures," as well as by X-ray therapy, avoiding unnecessary radiation to patients; and (3) the authorization for Doctors of Chiropractic to interpret their X-rays. (Submitted September 1975 and in similar language in June 1974.)

NATIONAL SPINAL HYGIENE FOUNDATION

Resolved that the ACA determine ways and means of establishing a national spinal hygiene foundation for the purpose of reaching the population with the facts of science upon which chiropractic is based and to provide a vehicle for public financial support for research and education within the profession. (Ratified by the House of Delegates June 1969.)

ORGANIZATION OF NATIONAL HEALTH SERVICES

(1) There should be a program for the expansion of group medical practice and HMO arrangements. (2) All supportive services (including laboratories, etc.) should be equally available to all licensed health-care providers without discrimination. (3) Federal law should provide for more effective assurance of national uniformity in Federal programs (such as Medicare and national health insurance), by (a) Federal licensing and standards for health-care intermediaries and carriers as a condition for serving in any Federal health-care or insurance program, and (b) Federal uniform standards of eligibility, coverage, utilization, etc., for all intermediaries or carriers in any Federal pro-

gram. (Guidelines for National Health Planning Goals, approved November 1975.)

PEER REVIEW APPEALS

The ACA Appeals Review Committee functions at the request of the carrier, attending physician, or the State Review Committee, only after the state or local committee has made the primary review, unless specifically requested by the State Review Committee, or upon failure of the State Review Committee to act within a reasonable period of time. (Approved July 1975.)

POINT OF ENTRY INTO NATIONAL HEALTH-CARE DELIVERY SYSTEM

Chiropractic is an initial point of entry or primary point of access for the health-care consumer. Because of its status as an independently licensed health-care profession and as an inescapable concomitant of the health-care consumer's freedom of choice, chiropractic must be an initial point of entry or primary point of access for the health-care consumer. Chiropractic serves as an alternative health-care service to medicine, and as such must be directly available to the consumer without prescription or required referral by any other health-care provider. The obverse obligation upon Doctors of Chiropractic, of course, is their referral to appropriate health-care providers of patients who come to them but are not suitable for chiropractic health care. (Guidelines for National Health Planning Goals, approved November 1975.)

PRACTICE AND PROCEDURES: FACILITIES

Resolved, that the House of Delegates reaffirm previous position by establishing that any and all facilities used by members of the chiropractic profession should meet jurisdictional licensing requirements for such facilities and that all practices and procedures used therein should be consistent with academics and clinical training in chiropractic colleges accredited by the accrediting agency of the Council on Chiropractic Education with reasonable scientific acceptability. (Ratified by the House of Delegates June 1975.)

PRACTICE MANAGEMENT COURSES

Resolved, that the House of Delegates of the American Chiropractic Association goes on record as endorsing only those practice building, practice promotion, practice management, and other related courses, lectures and/or services found acceptable to an Evaluation Committee appointed by the president subject to the approval of the House of Delegates and consistent with academics and clinical training in colleges having status with the Council on Chiropractic Education. (Ratified by the House of Delegates June 1975.)

PUBLIC AND PRIVATE HEALTH PROGRAMS

Resolved, that the ACA work for the inclusion of chiropractic in all public and private health programs by *name,* when possible. (Ratified by the House of Delegates June 1975.)

PUBLICATIONS, DRUGLESS HEALING

Resolved, that all tracts and brochures published by the ACA cease bearing statements that chiropractic is a drugless profession. (Ratified by the House of Delegates July 1974.)

PUBLIC HEALTH-CARE GOALS

It is the American Chiropractic Association's judgment that the primary and controlling consideration in any national health goals is the public interest of the consumers of health care and not the special interests of the providers of health care. The key issue should be what the public wants and needs . . . the Congress must itself decide on basic policies, practices and procedures, and not delegate them to private groups . . . In legislating on "health care," Congress is dealing with far more than the mere "professional practice of medicine."

We suggest that what some may regard as ". . . the professional practice of medicine . . ." is not the same as, nor necessarily conducive to, the best "health care" for the American people. The average American may not be an expert on medical practice but he is an expert on trying to obtain and to pay for health care. As providers for one form of health care, the chiropractic doctors of America believe that the interests of the health-care consumer, not those of the health-care provider, must be paramount in any national health planning and goals. (Guidelines for National Health Planning Goals, approved November 1975.)

PUBLIC HEALTH EDUCATION PROGRAM

The public's health depends in large measure on the public's knowledge of how each person individually can best help to protect and advance his own health and best make use of public and other facilities to this end. Therefore, effective national health goals must include a program of educating the general public concerning both preventive and remedial health care and concerning the best means to use all available services, both public and private. (Guidelines for National Health Planning Goals, approved November 1975.)

QUALITY HEALTH-CARE SERVICES

Chiropractic believes that protection of the public requires effective organization of a formal system, under public control, to monitor the quality, need for and the cost of health services provided to the public under national health insurance. Experience teaches that the services of a health-care professional can most effectively be reviewed by members of that profession itself.

We believe that it might also be fruitful to consider including consumer representation or participation in such review systems, not only for the protection of the quality of service but also to assure reasonable costs and to protect the public treasury . . .

It is appropriate, moreover, to note that a comprehensive program . . . would help to relieve the pressure on high-cost hospitalization by enabling patients to use, at their free choice, alternative services of lower-cost health-care providers for both preventative and therapeutic purposes. For example, an actual report . . . reported that these large insurance companies "detected no apparent increase in claim costs resulting from recognition of chiropractors . . ." . . . Various studies of state workmen's compensation programs . . . show a very much higher cost effectiveness in chiropractic as against alternative health-care benefits for substantially the same kind of illness . . .

In connection with protecting and advancing the quality of American health care, the ACA suggests the following considerations: (a) There should be a requirement of peer review on the quality of health care and a requirement of utilization review on the need of health care in all publicly sponsored and publicly supported health-care programs; (b) Peer review should be conducted by members of the specific profession being reviewed, provided however, that there should be . . . consumer participation mediaries quality evaluation; (c) Contract carriers or intermediaries in Federal programs should be required to establish and maintain effective quality and utilization control systems, on penalty of fines and disqualification; (d) In all Federally sponsored and Federally supported health-care programs, there should be a requirement for periodic license renewal of all participating health-care providers on the basis of regular continuing education programs or other evidence of maintenance of professional competency such as published research. In this connection, study should also be given to the wisdom and/or feasibility of requiring license re-examinations after some given period (such as 20 years) of practice; (e) There should be research and researcher-training programs in under-researched fields such as chiropractic; a broadening of training programs of specialized Federal health offices (such as the Bureau of Radiological Health), and an expansion of in-house research by NIH, VA, Armed Forces, etc., in under-researched areas such as chiropractic; (f) in all Federally sponsored and Federally supported health-care programs there should be a nondiscriminatory system of inclusion of all licensed health-care providers (including Doctors of Chiropractic) in all statistical reports and series, where relevant to public knowledge and the needs for quality and utilization control. (Guidelines for National Health Planning Goals, approved November 1975.)

SCOPE OF CHIROPRACTIC PRACTICE

Since the practice of chiropractic is regulated in all states, Puerto Rico, nine provinces in Canada, and a number of foreign countries, the present scope of practice is necessarily determined locally by existing statutory enactment and judicial determination in the separate jurisdictions. (ACA Master Plan, ratified by the House of Delegates June 1964, amended June 1975.)

SMOKING

Resolved, that the ACA in its combined professional opinion does hereby denounce cigarette smoking as a serious, multiple hazard to health and ACA dedicates itself to establishing a program of action designed to combat the dangers of and work toward the elimination of said hazard. (Ratified by the House of Delegates June 1969.)

Resolved, that the ACA support the surgeon general's findings that cigarette smoking is detrimental to the personal health of those who smoke, and the health of those nonsmokers within their smoky environment. (Ratified by the House of Delegates June 1972.)

Resolved, that the American Chiropractic Association shall state for the public record that it accepts the existing evidence that smoking is hazardous to the public's health. Resolved, that smoking is prohibited during official sessions of the House of Delegates. (Ratified by the House of Delegates June 1975.)

SPINAL HYGIENE

Resolved, that a vigorous program be instituted by the ACA for the dissemination of information as to the importance of the maintenance of a normally functioning spine and the necessity for early detection and correction of any problem that may develop. (Ratified by the House of Delegates July 1968.)

SUBLUXATION

The chiropractic use of the term "subluxation," in reporting, is usually valid as an objective descriptor, but is not acceptable as a diagnostic term, unless demonstrable as a scientifically acceptable and classified entity. The ACA recognizes and supports the consensus statement regarding subluxation approved and adopted by the profession at the Houston Conference of 1972. (Board approved July 1975.)

SUPPLY OF NATIONAL HEALTH SERVICES

In some respects, there is a shortage of health-care services and health-care facilities in many areas of the country, exacerbated by a maldistribution of available services and facilities and an overspecialization within them. Congress has shown an intensive desire to help solve the problem by expanding the availability of, at least, non-M.D. personnel. Therefore, it would fly in the face of Congressional purpose to exclude chiropractic from this effort. If the exclusion is based on a concern about chiropractic as such, the best way to meet such concern is not to ignore chiropractic, which will continue to serve millions of people, but rather to help rectify any alleged deficiencies so that chiropractic can do a better job within its legally authorized area of health care. The following considerations are submitted with respect to health manpower and facilities: (1) Federal support should be available for augmented education in all fields of state-licensed health-care professions which are recognized by the U.S. Office of Education for accreditation purposes, with guarantees of nondiscrimination against any licensed health profession; (2) There should be special incentives to universities for broadening their health-care education programs to encompass all officially recognized health programs (including chiropractic). Federal funds should be available for accredited chiropractic colleges equally with their availability for schools of medicine, nursing, etc.; (3) Federal scholarships for health-care education should require acceptance of the obligation by the beneficiary or recipient to serve, by assignment for limited periods of time, in underserviced areas at reasonable salaries. (Guidelines for National Health Planning Goals, approved November 1975.)

Uniform Licensure Legislation

Resolved, that the ACA recommend to each examining board and the Federation of Chiropractic Examiners standardized licensure legislation and universal acceptance of the National Board of Chiropractic Examiners. (Ratified by the House of Delegates July 1974.)

X-Ray, Chiropractic Objectives

It is recognized that roentgen rays are used by the health sciences for diagnostic or therapeutic purposes. The chiropractic profession utilizes X-ray only for diagnostic purposes and considers their use as one of the major diagnostic tools.

The ACA Commission on Insurance holds that there are two

facets to the responsibility of the chiropractic physician in the use of X-ray: (a) medical necessity for the radiation exposure to the patient; and (b) quality of studies consistent with scientific knowledge and acceptability. (Approved July 1975.)

X-RAY, DIAGNOSTIC

Roentgenology is one of the major diagnostic facets in the healing sciences and as utilized by chiropractic physicians is one of the major diagnostic tools of that science. Chiropractic does not use roentgenology or radiology therapeutically. The ACA supports the position of the Council on Roentgenology that declares the importance of diagnostic X-ray in the practice of chiropractic and the position of the Council that stresses the adherence to sound radiographic procedures. (Approved July 1975.)

X-RAY, FREE EXAMINATIONS

The ACA strongly condemns as unethical and dangerous the practice of advertising free spinal X-ray examinations and other indiscriminate uses of X-ray as a part of practice-building schemes and/or for other equally unethical purposes. (Approved 1967, reaffirmed 1972.)

X-RAY, PATIENT SAFEGUARDS

The chiropractic profession recognizes that diagnostic X-ray examinations, while offering inestimable benefits to the knowledge that is made available, have risks and possible detriments which must be weighed against those benefits. The ACA stands on record that there should always be clinical evidence of need for diagnostic X-ray examinations before such are performed. Use of X-ray as a routine procedure and from patients' self-referral is not good practice and is not condoned.

Proper measures of patient radiological protection including adequate collimation, filtration, gonadal shielding (when applicable) etc., should always be utilized. ACA admonishes all Doctors of Chiropractic to use all known measures of proper X-ray protection including proper selection of patients with due reference to age, childbearing status, and other factors, surely including clinical indication of need. Continuing education programs in radiological health and X-ray safety are and have been offered through the chiropractic colleges, state and national chiropractic association, and governmental agencies. The chiropractic profession has been among the leaders in the healing arts in participation in such courses and all D.C.s are urged to avail themselves of these. (Approved 1967, reaffirmed 1972.)

Reprinted, courtesy of the American Chiropractic Association, 2200 Grand Avenue, Des Moines, Iowa 50312

The Council on Chiropractic Education Position Paper

Reaffirmed and adopted at Las Vegas, Nevada, July 1, 1971.

The Council on Chiropractic Education, in recognition of its obligations to the public, the profession, and the scientific and educational community has adopted the following position:

1. Public

The Council on Chiropractic Education holds that it has a responsibility for the preservation and protection of the public health.

2. The Profession

The Council on Chiropractic Education holds that it has the responsibility to promote, establish, and maintain an academic environment which assures a qualitative educational program to provide graduates who will be ethical, competent, responsible, and professional Doctors of Chiropractic and thus insure perpetuation of chiropractic, as a disciplined member of the healing professions.

3. Scientific and Educational Community

The Council on Chiropractic Education holds that it has a responsibility to maintain standards of excellence so that it can best assist the rest of the scientific and educational world and to enhance the care of the sick alongside of the other healing professions.

4. The Individual Doctor of Chiropractic

The Council on Chiropractic Education holds that it has a responsibility to preserve for the Doctor of Chiropractic his rights as an independent practitioner in the healing arts in terms of the privileges defined by the individual state statutes; the equitable inclusion in all of the federal and state supported health programs, and insuring the perpetuity of the principles, traditions, and privileges of his profession.

5. Training-Education

While training is appropriate to vocational pursuits (auto mechanics, barbers, technicians, etc.), education is essential for those aspiring to become members of a profession. The Council on Chiropractic Education holds that education for those entering the healing-arts profession is doubly important. Conclusions, which are to be reached, based on the power to think connectedly, often have an effect upon life or death.

6. A Profession

The Council on Chiropractic Education holds to John Dale Russell's marks of a true profession and has the responsibility to preserve them within the chiropractic profession. The marks are:

a. A true profession attracts to its services people of excellent qualifications, with a superior level of intelligence, capable of being recognized as among the more substantial citizens of the community.

b. A true profession offers compensation that enables the one who follows it to live a good life, enjoy a good standard of living, and to contribute financially and otherwise to enterprises and activities that make for community improvement.

c. The practice of a true profession requires the exercise of independent judgment. The member of a profession is not just a hired hand.

d. The members of a true profession have considerable cohesiveness as a group usually within a national professional organization. They have a professional solidarity and mutual respect for other members of the profession.

e. A true profession is open only to those who have had extended scholarly preparation, specifically directed toward the type of work to be performed.

f. A true profession has a well-organized body of literature containing the principles, facts, and procedures related to its practice based upon science and not on individuals.

g. In a true profession there is usually an extensive research program for discovery and dissemination of new knowledge pertaining to the professional field and for the critical evaluation of old procedures.

h. A true profession lodges in its members considerable authority over the control of entrance into its calling. Some organized body within the profession sets up standards for entrance and sees that they are enforced.

i. A true profession offers a career. It is a life's work, affording opportunities for satisfying advancement within the profession itself.

j. A true profession has its own recognized code of ethics, either explicitly stated or so well understood by its members and the general public that it needs no formal statement. This code of ethics governs the members of the profession in all their activities.*

7. Two Years Preprofessional Education

The Council on Chiropractic Education holds a chiropractic

* J. D. Russell, College and University Business, Vol. 9, No. 1, July 1950, p. 17.

degree as being a first professional degree, as defined in HEW publication, requiring two academic years of pre-professional college education.

"First Professional Degree: A degree which signifies the completion of the academic requirements for selected professions based on programs which require at least two academic years of previous college work for entrance and which require a total of at least six years of college work for completion. Include dentistry, law, medicine, theology, veterinary medicine, etc."**

8. Intra-Institutional Relationship

The Council on Chiropractic Education, comprised of sister institutions with the common objective of educating Doctors of Chiropractic who are fully capable of assuming the responsibility of the preservation and restoration of the public health, demands that member institutions support The Council and each other with mutual respect and ethical deference.

9. Inter-Institutional Relationship

While The Council on Chiropractic Education encourages dialog and certain functional relationships with other institutions of higher education, it is fully aware that such relationships will not extend the institution's regional accreditation or federal acceptance to the chiropractic college, department or program.

"Because of the differing emphasis of the two types of accreditation, accreditation of the institution as a whole by a regional accrediting association should not be interpreted as being equivalent to specialized accreditation of each of the several parts of programs of the institution. Institutional accreditation does not validate a specialized program in the

** Education Directory, 1968–1969, Part 3, Page 458, U.S. Office of Education, Department of Health, Education, and Welfare.

same manner and to the same extent as specialized accreditation."***

10. Accreditation

Since the U.S. Office of Education or the National Commission on Accreditation does not accredit schools or colleges,
and since there is no accepted regional or professional accrediting agency charged with or structurally able to accredit
chiropractic colleges, The Council on Chiropractic Education has accepted its responsibility. The Council, because of
its continuous and documented history of operation in the
field of accreditation, its sets of standards in accord with the
criteria of the U.S. Office of Education, and its wide acceptance by the profession and outside agencies, will proceed
with its efforts for HEW acceptance as the chiropractic accrediting agency.

11. Research

Just as The Council on Chiropractic Education has a responsibility for education, it also has the responsibility of
encouraging and supporting research within its individual
institutions as well as in other institutions and agencies. The
Council holds that research is only valid and valuable when
conducted along accepted scientific methodology, with adequate records and controls, and by competent investigators.

12. Continuing Education

The Council on Chiropractic Education accepts its responsibility for postgraduate education for the profession. The
Council holds that only academic institutions can and
should conduct postgraduate courses and deplores the itinerant, privately conducted programs generally presented for
private gain.

The member institutions are charged with the responsi-

*** List of Nationally Recognized Accrediting Agencies and Associations,
Page 1, 1969 pamphlet issued by The Accreditation and Institutional Eligibility
Staff, U. S. Office of Education, HEW.

bility to conduct postgraduate courses that will keep the Doctor of Chiropractic abreast of recent advances.

13. Ethics

The Council on Chiropractic Education accepts its responsibility to enforce the ethics governing its member institutions and to promote the teaching and enforcement of professional ethics.

14. Quasi-Educational Institutions and Organizations

The Council on Chiropractic Education accepts its responsibility to encourage, aid, and develop academic excellence within and for the profession and the corollary responsibility of discouraging and utilizing every legal method to prevent the exploitation of education or training for personal gain whether in the form of itinerant courses, correspondence courses or substandard institutions which reflect discredit upon the profession. It is held that the proper education of a chiropractic physician complies with the high standards established by The Council, including two years of preprofessional college and four years of professional education.

Reprinted courtesy of the Council on Chiropractic Education, 2200 Grand Avenue, Des Moines, Iowa 50312

Bibliography

Books

Bach, Marcus. *The Chiropractic Story.* Los Angeles: DeVoss & Co., Inc., 1968.

Dintenfass, Julius. *Chiropractic: A Modern Way to Health.* New York: Pyramid Books, 1970.

Dye, A. August. *The Evolution of Chiropractic.* Richmond Hill, New York: Richmond Hill, 1969.

McClusky, Thorp. *Your Health and Chiropractic.* New York: Pyramid Publications, Inc., 1962.

Stanford Research Institute. *Chiropractic in California.* Los Angeles: The Haynes Foundation, 1960.

Magazines

The A. C. A. Journal of Chiropractic
Healthways Magazine

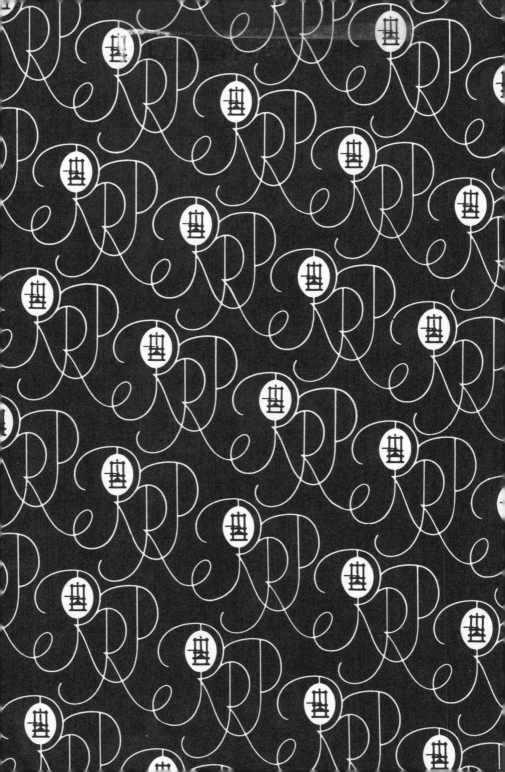